CASEY QUINLAN

Cancer For Christmas

**MAKING THE MOST
OF A
DAUNTING GIFT**

For Dave —
Live big, live
strong, live healthy.

the **Peppertree Press**

Sarasota, Florida

Casey
Quinlan

Cover Illustration by: Martha Gradisher
Book Design by: Elizabeth K. Peters

For information regarding permission,
Call 941-922-2662 or contact us at our website:
www.peppertreepublishing.com or write to:
the Peppertree Press, LLC.
Attention: Publisher
1269 First Street, Suite 7
Sarasota, Florida 34236

ISBN: 978-1-936051-41-0
Library of Congress Number: 2009933849
Printed in the U.S.A.
Printed August 2009

"Whether or not you know someone battling a "really big disease", this book has a gift for everyone: courage to dance with a life-threatening disease; laughter when least expected; and a gentle-but-firm kick in the pants toward taking the driver's seat of your own health and treatment options."

- **Mary Foley,**
author of *Live Like Your Nail Color*
Even If You Have Naked Nails

"Cancer for Christmas is a gift to anyone faced with the medical machine. Casey Quinlan's humor, irreverence, insight, and take-no-prisoners approach is an inspiration to anyone dealing with illness—or, for that matter, any major life challenge. You'll cry a little. You'll laugh a lot. And you won't be able to put this book down."

- **Shela Dean,**
Frequent Foreplay Miles,
Your Ticket to Total Intimacy

"Casey tells it like it is, which is exactlyhow she lives her life: full on, no holds barred! And now, thankfully, her honest words, wit, and wisdom will help women the world over realize that they can not only survive, but thrive! Thank you Casey for your inspiring story! You are truly a gift. XOXO!!"

- **Susie Galvez,**
international image consultant, speaker,
author, beauty industry expert and radio co-host of
"Girlfriend We Gotta Talk!"

*For anyone
who has ever heard a doctor
say something that
changed their life forever.*

Casey Quinlan

Foreword

I'm writing this book because somebody has to – there are eleventy-million-and-three books out there telling you that you can survive cancer. You certainly can, and I'm literal living proof. I don't need to add to that ever-growing pile.

I'd like to tell you the story about my cancer's detection and treatment, with the hope that you'll learn from my experience that yes, indeed, you can manage – survive? - cancer treatment.

Cancer treatment turns you into a patch of kudzu: first they cut you, then they poison you, then they burn you. Sometimes they poison you, burn you, cut you, and then poison you again. In some cases, they leave the poison on the shelf and just cut and burn you. Whatever horticultural-horror version of this metaphor you experience...you're kudzu.

The first time you hear "cancer" and your name used in a sentence you get a roaring sound in your ears. This prevents you from hearing much of what comes afterward, at least for a while. You sit there looking like a surprised cartoon character – at least that's what I felt like - every facial

feature frozen in a rictus of "say WHAT?"

That roaring sound dopplers in and out for a while, making it hard to hear what doctors are saying to you – and trust me, in today's drive-thru medical care, they don't say all that much, making hearing what they say critical. This makes it imperative for you to walk in either self-informed, or with a list of crisp interview questions that will get you up to speed on your situation, reveal actions to be taken, give you some idea if there's a Plan B, what to expect from any given decision, and so forth.

I boil it down to this: when you take your car to a car wash, do you want to go through inside the car, or strapped to the hood? Not being informed, not taking a proactive approach to your medical care, is like going through the car wash strapped to the hood. You'll wind up beaten to smithereens by the whirly-towel things, and get buckets of soap and wax up your nose, if you choose to go through the medical car-wash as an uninformed participant.

What follows is my story of getting cancer for Christmas in December 2007. At the time, it felt like the weirdest Christmas gift imaginable. Since then, I've come to truly see it as a gift.

It's a gift to me because it boiled down how I approach life to an essence - one that I savor daily. Hearing the word cancer and my name used in a sentence repeatedly both scared the **** out of me, and made me deeply grateful for every experience I had. Nothing like the specter of death to make you feel fully alive, as long as you manage to beat the Reaper. Eventually the Reaper wins, for all of us, but there's no reason to hurry up that process, is there? Life's too much fun, even in dark days, for me to want to shuffle off stage early.

And I hope it's a gift to you, one that will help you navigate the rapids of cancer treatment, or that you will use to help someone you love make decisions about their treatment. There can be dark days, as you navigate those rapids. Please feel free to laugh loud, to find the funny in those ridiculous situations (and positions!) you find yourself in – it'll keep you sane, and grounded, and in charge. It did that for me.

I'm not a doctor. I don't play one on TV. I haven't stayed in a Holiday Inn Express in ages. This book is not meant as a diagnostic tool, or any prediction of exactly what will happen to anyone post-diagnosis.

This is the story of my journey, the choices offered to me, and the research I did to learn the possible impact of each of those choices.

I'll share my research, my philosophical approach, and the reasons behind my decisions. I will not name the doctors in this story, since it's less important that I send you to specific *doctors than that I show you how to figure out if the doctor you're seeing is the right doctor for you.*

I've included blog posts and journal entries made during my trip through the cancer treatment car-wash, to give you an idea of what was going through my mind as I weighed treatment options. What I decided should not be adopted as a decision by anyone else – the decision-making process is what I'm trying to reveal, with the goal of helping anyone facing cancer, or an equally scary diagnosis, find a path to successful treatment that meets their needs.

And as a coda to each chapter, I've shared the gift I found in that part of the process – some of them surprising, some of them enlightening, all of them welcome.

ACKNOWLEDGEMENTS & THANKS:

Dr. DB, who diagnosed me early, and put me on the path to what I'm certain will be full recovery.

Dr. Randy B., whose input was critical, timely, and just right.

Dr. Sure Hands, whose delicate hands have treated me with the utmost care, and left very little trace of their work.

Dr. Cocktail, who continues to heal me, and in whose hands my long-term survival rests.

Dr. Glow Worm, who took good care of me in spite of the fact that she doesn't handle an angry patient well.

Dr. ESDP, who gave me the best Christmas gift I've ever gotten.

Crystal and Faith, who prove every day that oncology nurses are at the heart of healing cancer.

The Lymphedema Service at St. Mary's Hospital in Richmond, VA, for helping me manage my breast cancer souvenir.

Dr. Surgeon Ego & Dr. Drive-by, who gave me the low-bar measure for what I'll tolerate from a doctor who's treating me.

Mary, the original bodacious woman, who has been a rock throughout this journey. I'm livin' like my nail color, baby – Mammo Mango all the way!

Linda and Lyn, survivors who took me under their wing and helped ease my journey by sharing the story of theirs.

Donna, Dorothy, and Patricia, whose journeys were more terrifying than mine, and who kept me fearless.

Paula and Mort, who showed me what a cancer-fighting team looks like.

The women of ABWA's River City Express Network, whose concern and support have sustained me for years, including my most challenging one.

Terry, Susan, Mel, Kim, and all the women of Curves Short Pump, Curves Cross Ridge, and Curves Virginia Beach, who continue to throw me life-lines, and whose support is too deep and wide to measure.

Myra, who managed all the generosity that came my way.

The Greater Richmond Technology Council and The Venture Forum, whose leaders and membership kept my ship afloat, and continue to do so.

Linda, Kim, and Alicia, who love-bomb me constantly, and who gave me an iPod!

Carroll, who rode in on a white horse and swept me out of despair at exactly the right moment.

All my friends, each and every one of whom has lifted me up whenever my spirits sank.

All my clients, whose stories I tell with joy in my heart.

Hank, my very own Terminator, who is always there with just the right amount of whatever it is I need: bullets, Bordeaux, brandy, or just a willing ear.

And, as the last shall be first: my family, particularly Cece, without whom none of this would have been possible.

Chapter 1

I WANT MY MAMMO, MOMMA

I've always been a good little soldier about getting my mammograms. Started at 40 with my baseline, which is protocol for women who have no family history of breast cancer. I've made, and kept, my appointment every year, submitting to the tit-crusher without too much in the way of whining.

I even got a good comedy bit out of it, stating that you go in a 38C and come out a 44-Long, and when I get my hands on the sadistic bastard who invented this machine, I know just how I'll screen him for testicular cancer. The procedure does sort of beg for comic relief, and I was a stand-up comic in the '90s – low-hanging fruit like this is gold for a comedian, trust me.

This carried on for years. Make the appointment, get your boobs mashed flat, the doc says, "see you next year!" Fourteen years, to be exact.

I'd gotten cocky. Complacent, even. I'd rescheduled my 2007 mammogram twice, when what seemed to be more important appointments created a conflict.

I presented myself for my fifteenth mammogram on the morning of Monday, December 10, 2007, at the offices of Dr. DB, where I'd been going for mammograms since 2000. They were busy, things took a bit longer that usual, and I had a meeting later that morning to pick up a payment from a client.

Important stuff. Let's hurry this up, huh?

I finally got myself mashed, then got dressed to talk to Dr. DB in what had become our annual "no change, see you next year" 60-second conversation".

Here is the first piece of practical advice I have for you: when mammograms are a part of your life, find an imaging center where you look at your films with the doctor. There are two imaging centers where I live (in Richmond, Virginia) that do this. After my first seven years of boob-mashing, when I still lived in New York, which were followed up weeks later with a "you're OK" letter, discovering that it was possible to know before you walked out that all was well was a welcome change.

So, I went into Dr. DB's office, the Kingdom of the Light Box, with my films – and after 15 years of mammograms, that's a lot of films – up all around the light box walls. There they were, "the girls", lit up from all sides, each view looking essentially the same, year after year.

Cancer For Christmas

This year's models were on the box next to his desk. I walked in, we walked over to the films, and at the same moment, we both leaned over and said, "What's THAT?"

"That", in this instance, being a tiny spot in the lower midline of my left breast. A spot that had never been there before.

Dr. DB said he wanted to do a magnification mammogram, and maybe an ultrasound. I said I had a busy morning, and would come back later in the week.

As I dashed out of the office, I stopped at the desk and made said appointment for Thursday, Dec. 13. When I left, I took with me a nagging little voice saying, "What IS that?"

The next few days were busy. I work with the Technology Council in Richmond, and that Wednesday they held a summit conference on IT in healthcare – irony is one of my very favorite things – and I spent several minutes talking to a doctor, Randy B., one of the experts in healthcare IT presenting at the summit.

Remember him, he'll show up again soon.

Thursday morning, one of my presentation-coaching clients was speaking at an accounting & finance forum breakfast. During our work together over the previous ten days, I'd learned that she was a breast cancer survivor. I didn't mention my funky mammogram, but thought that if I needed some advice, I'd ask her for recommendations.

After watching her nail her presentation, and get mobbed afterward by CFOs (chief financial officers) and CEOs who wanted to talk about doing business - I love it when a plan comes together - I headed back to the imaging center. Telling myself all the way there that this nagging little voice, the "what IS that?" voice, should just shut the **** up.

The magnification mammogram of the left boobular area took less than five minutes. I'd been told that an ultrasound would be next, but after the technician took the films to the doctor, she came back in and said there'd be no ultrasound. The doctor wanted to see me.

Somehow, this was not reassuring.

I went into the Kingdom of the Light Box, where the doctor and I stood before the magnification films. He wanted to do a biopsy on whatever-it-was, which through magnification looked – duh – much bigger.

He kept saying that there was no reason to worry, that most of the biopsies he did turned out to be benign, that only 30% came back as cancer, blah, blah, blah.

I didn't really hear what he was saying. I was too busy staring at the image, remembering all the medical stories I'd been a part of in my days in network news.

Cancer For Christmas

"Irregular star pattern. And those sure look like spicules to me."

I didn't say it out loud, but I was now starting to have that feeling you get when you're watching a suspense movie, and some poor fool is about to get done in by the bad guy.

Cue the scary music.

The biopsy was scheduled for Wednesday, Dec. 19.

I spent the next 18 hours in a quiet mental riot. What if it WAS cancer? I had medical insurance through my almost-ex-husband's company, but the financial agreement we'd forged when separating in early 2006 was about to end, meaning that a significant portion of my income was about to dry up. If I wound up with cancer, how would I be able to work on business development for Mighty Casey Media?

Dammit, I didn't have TIME for cancer – my schedule was full!

I had just, for the first time, drawn up a soup-to-nuts annual plan, with the help of my Mastermind group. The ink was drying on what looked to be a meaningful step toward getting back on my feet financially, with some audacious-yet-achievable goals for 2008.

Cancer was most definitely not in that plan.

The morning of Friday, Dec. 14, I had a meeting with that Mastermind group. I had trouble sleeping the night before – gee, I wonder why? – and was still in something of a swivet as I drove to the meeting.

Suddenly, I was hit with a moment of clarity.

Luckily, it wasn't accompanied by the sound of a car crash, because to say I was distracted would be putting it (very) mildly.

That clarity – a small, clear voice that was my own – said this: whatever "it" was, cancer, a cyst, or nothing at all, "it" represented all the anger, all the resentment, all the crap I'd collected in my 55 years on the planet.

"It" was going to be removed, and I would move on, completely free.

BLOG POST 12/14/2007

I'll Kick Its Ass, Baby!
Found out yesterday that I might have breast cancer. Will know next Thursday, after a biopsy on Wednesday. The best part of this whole thing is that, after struggling yesterday to figure out what the message was from this, the message became clear: the tissue that will be removed, whatever it is, will be a complete encapsulation all the anger, resentment, self-doubt, self-abnegation...in fact, all the **** collected over 55 years on planet Earth.

That's the definition of a win, at least in my book.

Cancer For Christmas

Cancer? If it is, I'll kick it's A**, baby.

Arriving at that conclusion was a turning point for me, and not just in how I was going to deal with the immediate future of biopsy-and-whatever-came-after. I really did feel as though I was getting the chance to move past all the "stuff" I'd collected in a lifetime that included two failed marriages, more disappointments than I could shake any kind of stick at, and a lingering sense that I still hadn't figured out what I wanted to be when I grew up.

I've joked for years about the emotional baggage we all collect over a lifetime – what I refer to as "my full set of Samsonite." I felt, with this epiphany, as though I was being presented with an opportunity to strip down all the crap, to jettison what wasn't serving me, to move into a freer, happier way of being.

That full set of Samsonite was reduced to the size of a small shadow in my left breast. Whatever else it was, it was my chance to reassess my baggage, and leave anything unnecessary at the side of the road.

It was outta here. All of it.

I spent the six days between magnification mammogram and biopsy searching with my fingers in the area shown on the film, and all the other parts of my breasts, for any sort of lump. There wasn't one. The only thing I found was the bruising that showed up due to my relentless searching.

Take that as a warning: no palpable lump does not mean you don't have to go for a mammogram. On the other hand, if you DO feel a lump, get thee to a mammogram as fast as you possibly can. The key here is early detection – cancer found in the early stages, Stage I or Stage II, is much more survivable than it is if it gets to Stage III. At Stage IV, you're literally in a fight for your life.

I presented myself at the imaging center on Wednesday morning, Dec. 19, for my biopsy.

BLOG POST 12/19/2007

OK, That Was Fairly Weird

...my biopsy, I mean.

On the weirdness scale, it ranks somewhere between sedation dentistry and getting hit in the head with a two-pound sledgehammer..

I really could have done without the show & tell after the procedure. Somehow, seeing the size of that freakin' needle - needle? More like a rocket launcher! - did NOT make me feel better. That, and the fact that the tissue-remover deal sounded just like my electric toothbrush. Oh, GREAT - now I'll have flash-backs while brushing my teeth.

My dentist will be so very pleased. I mean, to me all dentists wind up looking like Laurence Olivier in "Marathon Man" anyway, so this is NOT a good thing.

Results tomorrow.   Stay tuned...

I recommend that, should you find yourself in the same time-for-your-biopsy-Mrs.-Johnson boat, you take an iPod loaded with Soundgarden, the Ramones, Pearl Jam, Nine Inch Nails, and Wagner's Götterdämmerung, the better to drown out the sound of projectiles being fired into your boob, repeatedly, in service of grabbing and grinding up shreds of tissue to ship off to the pathology lab. I did not have said iPod, and deeply regretted its absence.

Lashings of lidocaine meant that this procedure wasn't particularly painful – other than the vise that twisted my breast around to the point that I felt like saying, "Hey, it's not a faucet, guys!" Definitely tit-in-the-wringer time.

There's also the highly amusing position one finds oneself in – lying facedown on a table with your boob dangling down through a hole.

Twisting, banging, and grinding complete, I was asked to return the following afternoon for the results.

I, of course, spent a very restful night (not), thinking not at all about the following day (ha!), and sleeping the sleep of babies.

Fat chance.

BLOG POST 12/19/2007

In the Spirit of the Season, as a Celt

...which season I identify as Yule, I offered the following toast at a gathering here in RVA last night.

There were stares. And then there were cheers, even from the avowed Baptists:

In the northern latitudes, my ancestral place, the winter solstice marked the end of the reign of darkness and the promise of the rebirth of the sun. As Christianity spread to Scandinavia and the British Isles, Christmas celebrations supplanted Solstice Night. However, I choose to celebrate as my ancestors did, to celebrate the end of darkness - death - and the birth of new light - life.

Tomorrow, I will learn if I have breast cancer.

Under the mistletoe, allheal, the plant of peace, I celebrate the end of personal darkness. The release and removal of all old anger, past resentment, lingering self-doubt, all the crap collected on a 55-year journey. Tonight, I acknowledge the darkness. And I turn toward the light.

I honor the rebirth of me.

Cancer For Christmas

Whatever comes to pass in the current dances-with-my-left-boob, I will emerge stronger, better, and unbowed.

I wish ME joy. And I wish joy for all of you. Raise your glasses to the end of darkness, and the coming of the light. Whatever happens, this feels like the best Yule ever. Or Christmas. Whatever.

––––––––

I was terrified, but I was determined not to let terror get the best, or even the better, of me. I don't consider myself particularly brave, but one of my core philosophies is that when you face a big problem, you can either scream about it, or start dealing with it.

If you scream, you waste time and breath. Screaming does nothing for you, and it sure doesn't do much for anyone within ear-shot, either. Plus, you just wasted all that time on screaming that could have been better spent looking for ways to solve the problem.

Denial doesn't work very well either, particularly in situations like this. Worst-case scenario was: I have cancer. However, if I did have cancer, it looked like it had been detected early, making my long-term survival probability pretty good. Denial – also known as running away – wouldn't do anything positive for my survival percentage. In fact, running away would likely kill me.

Even with all the struggles I had been through in the last few years, I enjoyed my life much too much to be willing to give it up.

So, I cowgirled up and kept moving forward.

The Gift

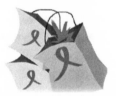

Discovering the capacity for meaningful change with an epiphany about the "stuff" we all haul around — you can only really fly when you let go.

Chapter 2

CANCER FOR CHRISTMAS

The next day passed about as quickly as any day can when you're counting down to a 2:30pm revelation that your life literally hinges on. Time slowed to the point that it seemed the clock was moving backwards.

I left the house around 1pm, on the theory that getting out and moving around would help distract me. I headed to a local grocery store that has a terrific deli and salad bar, and as I was walking past the checkout lines, I saw a familiar face.

Dr. Randy B., who I'd met at the healthcare IT summit a week ago, was there, with his wife, buying groceries.

Now, don't ask me why this guy, whose practice is miles away to the south, and who lives miles away to the west, was buying groceries near my house on this particular day, at exactly this time, other than that he was supposed to run into me.

I said hello, he introduced me to his wife, and asked what I was up to. I replied that I was killing time until I could find out if I had cancer.

He goggled at me, and then said to let him know what I found out. I said I would, and we parted ways.

I ate lunch, tried to read a magazine, and eventually it was time to go get the news, whatever it turned out to be.

When I got to the imaging center, I wondered if I was imagining things when it seemed that the nurse who took me back to the consultation room was being extra solicitous. Is she being super-nice because…I HAVE CANCER???

I shoved that thought aside, and waited for the doctor. He came in, and I said,"let's cut to the chase – what is it?"

"Cancer."

I guess the nurse DID know.

Oh, boy. I got cancer for Christmas. Now that's a booby prize.

I guess I've got more anger and resentment that has to be removed?

I didn't hear much of what he said after "cancer" – when you hear that word and your name in a sentence, that roaring sound I mentioned earlier drowns out everything else, as your brain skids around screaming,

Cancer For Christmas

"HOLY ****! AM I GONNA DIE? WTF?" and other calming, quieting thoughts.

I then went down the assembly line, collecting referrals and appointments with the surgeon that Dr. DB sends his breast cancer diagnoses to. I found myself out in the parking lot, headed to the gym, with the roaring sound in my ears starting to fade.

My brain was still screaming "HOLY ****!" – but I was trying to put one foot in front of the other. Standing still wasn't possible right now.

I called my almost-ex-husband who, in his usual glass-completely-empty-and-smashed-on-the-floor way, had me trying to cheer HIM up while I shared my newly minted cancer status. As I sat in my car outside the gym, it felt like I couldn't string two thoughts together. There was a giant boulder the size of Table Mountain in my head, with I'VE GOT BREAST CANCER scrawled across it in letters twenty feet high. It was now about 5pm, and I was in a fog, trying to figure out what to do.

I tried working out, but my heart (and mind, and all other parts) weren't really in it. As I left the gym, I called my friend Mary. I asked her where she was, and it turned out she was at a gourmet store around the corner from my house. I said, "wait there!" and drove over, where we met up in the parking lot. I told her my news. She immediately said that I had to come over to her house. She and the man she calls Crazy Glue (he's crazy about her, she's stuck on him), were having a dinner party, and I needed to be there.

I wasn't sure I wanted to be around a bunch of people, particularly people I didn't know, but Mary talked me into coming by for a drink, since it appeared that I clearly needed one. Plus, Crazy Glue – Bill - is a terrific cook.

That evening was another of the gifts I got that day, the first being the chance encounter with Dr. Randy B. One of Mary & Bill's neighbors, Carol, listened to me talk about my interesting Christmas present, then jumped up and ran out the door. She was back in seconds, holding a pile of booklets and brochures from Genentech, the pharmaceutical company. She had just started volunteering with the Susan G. Komen Foundation chapter in Richmond. Said booklets and brochures were a road map to navigating breast cancer diagnosis and treatment that she'd gotten at a training session that very week.

How to read a pathology report, questions to ask, what staging was, the whole nine yards.

Armed with that, and basking in the glow of the love of friends and some really outstanding food – lamb Wellington. Who knew? - I headed home with the feeling that whatever was on tap, I'd be up to the challenge.

I hoped.

Cancer For Christmas

BLOG POST 12/20/2007

I'm Reminded of a Favorite Jules Pfeiffer Cartoon ...wherein the guy ponders all the things in his life that cause cancer – the most recent report held that scotch was a terrible carcinogen – so he lifts a glass (scotch, of course) and declares, "Whoopee! Cancer!"

I'm here to tell you that I have reason to say the same thing. I learned today that I have breast cancer.

It was discovered in my routine annual mammogram, it has not even achieved palpable-lump status, and by all accounts (so far) I'm looking at a lumpectomy and a round of radiation.

Biopsy pathology report: Invasive ductal adenocarcinoma, grade II lesion.

In English, that means I have breast cancer.

Whoopee! Cancer!

Good news is that it was discovered by my annual (always routine before!) mammogram. Bad news is...well, it's CANCER, dammit.

Now I'm trying to research the surgeon that I've been referred to - why isn't there a consumer reports site for doctors? That would make sense, but...like so much that makes sense, at least to me, it doesn't exist. Or, if it does, it isn't easy to find.

Stay tuned...

Whatever happens, I will be 100% fine.

Journal entry 12/20/07

Pissed off.

I blew right past denial and shock, went straight for the rage. Not surprising, really, considering that I've defaulted toward anger most of my life.

In my teens and twenties, I was repeatedly adjured against being pissed off – not "nice". I learned to temper my temper, although the usual cause for what I was feeling was much less temper than a deep desire to change something I found unacceptable.

Well, I've got early stage breast cancer, and I find that both unacceptable and a fact of life. I don't think that being pissed off is necessarily a bad thing in this situation, since I'd rather roar than cry. I'm weird that way.

The thing that scares me most? Not physical stuff, like boob whacking (although I don't think I'm facing that). Money. I have no cash. I haven't had anything like enough to pay the bills for a while, and I'm wondering how I'm going to change that.

I default toward get-it-spend-it, which leads to where I'm at right now. I have a lot to offer, but I'm not at all sure how to turn that into gelt. And if I get said gelt, will I be able to hang on to any of it?

In other words…WTF on a universal scale.

––––––––––

I had been terrified since the magnification mammogram revealed something that appeared to have an irregular star pattern and spicules. Now I had a focus for my terror – a confirmed cancer diagnosis. That night, I got my first taste of what would ultimately be the magic elixir that got me through this whole medical-car-wash ordeal: the unwavering support of friends. Even people I didn't know, or know well, would, over the next several months, do and say things that smoothed my path, that calmed my fears, that eased my mind.

The best way to manage treatment is with clarity of mind and purpose. Everyone who reached out and helped me gave me that in spades.

Here's a very important message – share your story, what's happening with your medical situation, with your friends. If you need help, ask. If you need support, ask. Asking for help will get you help – sometimes from surprising sources, and in totally unexpected ways.

Build a support network, and rely on it during treatment. If your family can't deal with what's going on, find a support group or make one of your own out of fellow patients or friends.

You're in the fight of your life – don't accept anything less than everything you need. If you have financial challenges, which I most certainly did, reach out – in your community and online. There are lots of non-profit organizations dedicated to helping people in their fight against life-threatening diseases, and many of them have patient advocates who help identify financial resources.

Get what you need to survive. Don't settle for less.

The Gift

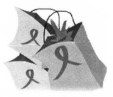

Always share your challenges, always ask for help – it will arrive. Your openness will inspire an open heart in others.

Chapter 3
SURGEON SURGERY

I sent Dr. Randy B. an email before I went to bed the day I got cancer for Christmas, asking him who he'd want operating on his wife or his sister if they had breast cancer. The next morning, he replied with the name of "the boob man of Richmond", as well as a strong recommendation that I contact Dr. Sure Hands, a young woman surgeon who he said was developing a great reputation in breast surgery.

I also sent a message to my breast cancer survivor client, the one I had worked with just a week previously, to find out what she recommended. As someone who'd been-there-done-that, I hoped she could give me some input that would help me arrive at a decision. She told me that her doctor had been "the boob man of Richmond", who had also treated another of my colleagues who had fought breast cancer the previous year.

Dr. DB's office had made an appointment with their pet surgeon for Wednesday, Dec. 26. I called "the boob man of Richmond" that Friday, Dec. 21 to inquire about an appointment – he couldn't see me until February.

I thought that might be a little long to wait – if I was having trouble sleeping now, I could only imagine how bad it would get if I had to wait more than a month to see what would happen next. Plus, I wanted this thing growing in my left breast outta there. I called Dr. Sure Hands and, sure enough, she could see me on Christmas Eve, the following Monday.

That gave me the weekend to develop a set of surgeon interview questions that would put me in the Katie Couric/Mike Wallace category for penetrating inquiry.

Using the Genentech literature as a starting point, and assembling more data and detail from BreastCancer. org, Cancer.org, and a guy I like to call Dr. Google, I had enough questions for a half-hour documentary with no commercial breaks.

I arrived at Dr. Sure Hands' office the afternoon of Christmas Eve clutching a legal pad with a list of questions that would impress the writer of a Vanity Fair profile.

CASEY'S SAMPLE DOCTOR Q&A – LATHER, RINSE, REPEAT AS OFTEN AS NECESSARY

Given this diagnosis, what treatment options would you suggest?

Cancer For Christmas

In your experience, statistically how many patients are lumpectomy candidates and how many mastectomy, with my same circumstances?

What's your approach with a lumpectomy?

What's your approach with a sentinel-node biopsy?

What type of marker do you use to identify the sentinel nodes?

How long does the surgery typically take?

What's the recovery process like?

How often have you discovered that a mastectomy was necessary, when you had planned a lumpectomy?

What's the process with an axial excision, if you find out that's necessary?

What kind of complications can arise with a lumpectomy?

With a mastectomy?

With an axial excision?

Who decides on radiation and/or chemo?

What's the treatment for hormone-positive cancer?

What's the treatment for HER2-positive cancer?

Who would you recommend as an oncologist?

Who would you recommend as a radiation oncologist?

The first thing that told me I was going to like Dr. Sure Hands: when I was taken back to the exam room, I immediately started to peel off my clothes. The nurse said not to do that yet, since Dr. Sure Hands would come in to talk to me first, and then she would do the exam after we had had a chance to talk.

There's a distinct power shift that happens when you're naked, and the other person in the room is not. They've got all the cards, and you feel like something that's been judged and found wanting. To have a first meeting with a surgeon with at least the appearance that doctor and patient are on an equal footing felt revolutionary, and very welcome, to me.

When I left, I knew that I was an ideal lumpectomy candidate, what steps were involved in the surgery, and in surgery prep. I'd arrive at the hospital, get shot up with blue dye to light up my lymph nodes, have something called a 'needle loc', and then on to surgery. They'd take two or three sentinel nodes, get an immediate pathology report on those, and then either do an axial excision (full removal of nodes at the underarm), or button me up. Then the tumor would be removed, with 360° of surrounding tissue, and sent off for a full pathology assay.

Based on how surgery went, and the final pathology report, I'd know what the next steps might be, if chemotherapy was on my radar, and what sort of radiation protocol I'd have.

Cancer For Christmas

There's a great new radiation treatment called Mammo-Site, where a small balloon device is placed in the tumor site, and radiation treatment is delivered directly to the area where the tumor was, the tumor bed. The radiation itself takes only five days, which is markedly less than the five to eight weeks of traditional radiation treatment for breast cancer.

Stay tuned to find out which type of radiation treatment I had – sometimes choices are made for us as a situation unfolds, which you can't predict ahead of time!

Also, for anyone wondering if I ever considered alternative, non-surgical treatment to surgery – no. I do believe that alternative medicine has a lot to offer, but in this case, I was going the traditional route. I trusted this surgeon, and I had many friends who had been treated for breast cancer – all of them had elected surgical tumor removal. I was stickin' with the group.

BLOG POST 12/26/2007

In our last episode, our heroine bemoaned the lack of easily accessible consumer data on surgeons.

Turns out that in the surgery game – just like in any business – referrals are key. However, one learns quickly that one needs to consider the source (now there's a news flash, right?) when evaluating the referral.

Bottom line, I'm being a chauvinist. Grrl parts = grrl doctor.

I've found a terrific woman who makes me feel like I'm in great healing hands. So I'm booked for surgery on Jan. 14.

I was only half-kidding about the female-chauvinist remark. No one knows better than another woman how important body image is to a female. I'm no show-stopper, at least not any more, but it's important when I look in the mirror that I look like me. Dr. Sure Hands clearly understood that, and made it clear that she did during our discussion. She never pushed away a question, never rushed through an explanation, and never finished a meeting with me until she knew that I understood everything that was going to happen.

Well, there was one minor point, one that's dealt with in the next chapter, but that ultimately led to more comedy than rage. Stay tuned for that story.

What, you might ask, happened with the OTHER surgeon, the one my radiologist referred me to?

Dr. Surgeon Ego is the name I gave him.

At a minimum, you have to be able to tolerate someone who's going to be using a scalpel on your soft parts. At least I do. And this was, after all, happening to me.

Bottom line, the guy was a jerk.

Cancer For Christmas

From the moment I was told to strip to the waist before he arrived on the scene (see previous comments about the power trip inherent there), to him doing everything short of patting me on the head and calling me "little lady" when he did arrive, and especially including the moment when, after he asked what I did and I told him I helped companies tell their stories, the son of a bitch laughed at me, I knew this guy and I were not going to be seeing each other again.

I'm sure if you asked him, he'd deny that he was laughing AT me…but I've got a pretty thick skin. And I know the difference.

I ran down my questions, but sensed that Dr. Surgeon Ego wasn't really interested in answering questions. He was all about making sure that I understood that he was a surgeon, he did this all the time, it was no big deal, trust him.

Dr. Sure Hands won hands down over Dr. Surgeon Ego. Pun fully intended.

The good news is that the Dr. Surgeon Ego type is disappearing like the dinosaurs they are – we can speed their departure by refusing to play along. Don't stick with a doctor who doesn't communicate with you, or who doesn't treat you like a partner in your quest for health. Male or female, give the jerks the shove.

JOURNAL ENTRY 12/26/2007

OK, I found a surgeon. Of course, it's a girl – was there even a question? Of course (again), I saw a traditional-dude-surgeon today, who made a few comments about "general surgeons" that had me almost second-guessing myself...but then I woke up. Traditional-dudes are so 20th century. Paternalistic jackass-ery is not healing in any way, at least not for me.

I'm stickin' with the grrl. Who will heal me.

The Gift

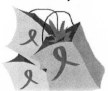

Curiosity + Research = Great Questions.
Always ask questions when you're a
stakeholder in the outcome – and make sure
you understand the answers.

Chapter 4

LET ME OUTTA HERE!

As part of the preparation for surgery, Dr. Sure Hands sent me for a breast MRI. During the scheduling session, when we set up everything from the MRI through the surgery itself, I was asked if I was claustrophobic.

I knew why they were asking – MRIs happen in small tubes – and I said no, I wasn't. I am, among many other things, a scuba instructor. I've taught numerous people how to manage the claustrophobic feelings that can arise when putting on scuba gear, particularly a mask, for the first time.

I lived to regret saying no to that question.

The MRI was booked for the morning of Jan. 3, 2008. I arrived at the imaging center, which was far enough south of my house in central Virginia that I thought I might be in North Carolina, and I was the first vict… um, patient, through the door that day.

I was taken back to a changing room, and told to strip to the waist and put on a short gown. The technician came to retrieve me, and in we went to face the MRI god.

I knew immediately that there might be a problem.

First, there was a bizarre looking contraption attached to the table that had two little round holes in it. Yes, those were little trap doors for my boobs.

I was told to lie face down on the table, with my boobs in the trap door apertures, and my arms up in diver position. A mass of pillows was placed under my head, since there was a big gap between the trap-door add-on and my head.

The tech hooked me up to an IV that would administer light-up-my-soft-parts dye, the better to see inside the boobular area(s). I was given a stern admonition that any moving around or deep breathing on my part would mean that we'd have to start the procedure all over again, and then she mashed several heavy blankets on top of my head and shoulders, "to keep me warm".

Houston, we now had a very big problem.

I was face down in a mass of pillows, with my arms out past my head in diver position. I now had a big wad of blankets on top of my head, and I was shoved down into a squeezy tube about an inch wider than my shoulders.

Cancer For Christmas

I couldn't breathe! I felt like McMurphy being suffocated by Chief Bromden in "One Flew Over the Cuckoo's Nest", and I could tell that my blood pressure was jacking up enough to give me a vascular lobotomy.

Can you say…CLAUSTROPHOBIA?

I had occasion during the next 45 minutes to reflect on how much I appreciate meditation and yoga. Those two disciplines allowed me to not freak out and shoot my way out of the place.

As I listened to the incessant banging that's the central feature of MRI imaging – in addition to claustrophobia - rising in pitch and frequency, then falling, then rising again, I thought to myself that this was exactly the sort of opera that Phillip Glass would compose if he was piss-drunk and high on acid. This may not seem a comforting thought to you, but trust me – when you're suffocating, finding something to amuse yourself with is critical.

Apparently, my close-to-madness discomfort didn't translate into any problems getting the MRI to completion. In fact, the tech said I had, and I quote, "been AWESOME."

Yoga, meditation, and Monty Python – the trinity of mental stability under duress, I guess.

JOURNAL ENTRY 1/3/08

Still pissed off, but less so. Anger is entirely focused on this 'thing' inside my left breast, and that focus is all about 'get it OUT'.

The next time someone asks me if I'm claustrophobic, I'll have to answer "no...except for MRIs". Holy ****.

I almost had a stroke in that thing. Had I been on my back, I don't think it would have been any kind of scary, but with my head smashed into pillows – that were supposed to make me comfortable, but instead made me feel like I was suffocating – and my arms over my head, the entire process seemed designed to make one feel as if one was drowning. If not for yoga breathing and meditation experience, I woulda shot my way outta there. Holy ****.

So then, I went for my pre-op poke-n-prod at the hospital, and my BP was jacked. I said, "OK. Let's review. For the last couple of weeks, my name and cancer have regularly appeared in the same sentence. I had an MRI today that almost killed me. Now I'm in a hospital setting, with all the lovely fluorescent lights, surrounded by people in white coats. AND I HAVE WHITE-COAT SYNDROME. What do YOU think is jacking my BP??" They left me alone for a while, and it was down 40 points. I rest my case.

Cancer For Christmas

New rule to live by: when they say MRI, ask for some valium, and have someone drive you home from the imaging center. Even if you've never been claustrophobic in your life, when you find yourself having a face-down-mashed-into-pillows-can't-breathe MRI, the situation might just turn you into a whimpering infant. It did that to me.

The MRI was the last step before surgery. One of the things I realized as I counted down to S-for-Surgery Day was that I needed an advance directive. I wasn't really worried that Dr. Sure Hands and her team would do me any irreparable harm while excising the cancer from my left breast, but as a former Girl Scout, "be prepared" still sound like words to live, or die, by. The part where I wind up in a persistent vegetative state, tied to a ventilator with no hope of recovery, is to be avoided at all costs. I needed that in writing.

I spent New Year's Eve in the hills of western Virginia with a friend. He and I had spoken many times, in a general way, about end-of-life issues. We'd made a fist-bump deal that he'd stand on my breathing tube, and I'd do the same for him, should the need arise.

It was time to formalize that fist-bump deal.

Before I headed out to his place, I downloaded an advance directive written for the state of Virginia, inserting my name and his in the appropriate squares. We spent part of New Year's Eve morning at his bank, getting the copies signed and notarized.

He came down to the flatlands of Richmond, joining my sister and me for a "condemned woman eats a hearty meal" dinner the night before surgery.

He would also stay on until I was sprung from the hospital, ready to step in waving the advance directive should the worst-case scenario come to pass. It was around this time that he started referring to himself as my Terminator, which he still does.

The one-and-only rule my friend imposes when visiting the flatlands is that oysters be on the menu. We found a place in Shockoe Bottom that had not only oysters, but also all-you-can-eat snow crab legs. The condemned woman watched as her designated plug-puller pulled the plug on a couple dozen oysters and what were ultimately too-numerous-to-count amounts of snow crab legs.

Feeling that she might live to regret such a Lucullan feat of ingestion just prior to surgery, our heroine got outside a salad and grilled fish, washed down with just the right amount of wine.

And then headed home to get very little sleep at all, which had become an unhappy habit over the last month.

The Gift

Learning to take the steps necessary to preserve your dignity, and your choices.

Chapter 5

FIRST, THEY CUT YOU
(THE FIRST CUT IS THE DEEPEST)

5:00am is bloody early.

Truly the ass-crack of dawn.

It was also the hour of reveille on the morning of surgery, and of course I didn't really need the alarm clock. I hadn't slept more than a couple of hours at a stretch for a month, since the original funky mammogram.

Off we went in the darkness to see what a lumpectomy really involved.

I checked in at the ambulatory surgery center, and was sent to nuclear medicine for the injection of blue dye that would light up the sentinel lymph nodes. I wound up feeling sorry for the poor bastard who shot me up – the injection was so painful, I stuffed a pillow into my mouth so I could scream without having security burst into the room to see who was being murdered.

I went back to the waiting room, and after a while I was invited to visit mammography. Oh, boy – another tit-crushing!

They grabbed, literally, an image of my left breast, and I was invited to lie face-down on yet another table with a cute little trap door in it for my left boob.

Then a doctor came in and shoved a long, thin needle into my boob. This is called "needle localization", or "Spanish Inquisition needle-jabbing procedure", whichever works best for you.

I do believe that medical professionals are under the impression that there are no nerves in breast tissue. Here's a news flash, team: YES, THERE ARE. Lidocaine works. I suggest using it.

Heads up, all you medical professionals – it may be just another procedure for you, but it's the only one your patient is having today, or maybe in this lifetime. Remember that, and act accordingly. Don't just jab us and run. If the roles were reversed, how would YOU like to be treated? All we ask is that you not treat us like a piece of meat.

Now all that remained was the actual surgery. I was taken into a prep room where I stripped down, put on the always stylish gown, and was hooked up to an IV.

There was an ever-increasing parade of nurses, technicians, doctors, orderlies, and I think I even saw a partridge in a pear tree and Waldo at one point. I can't be certain, because by now some blessed member of the parade had administered something"to relax me". Whoever did that earned my undying gratitude.

I then became the focal point of a procession of medical personnel as I was wheeled into the OR. By now, I was entertaining the troops with my scintillating observations about what was going on (wow, lotta people work in this hospital, don't they?) and how I was feeling (wow, I haven't been this high since I was in college in the Haight Ashbury in the'70s!)

Then the lights went out.

I woke up in the recovery room, and saw a wall clock that indicated it was 12:30pm. Doing a fuzzy-brained calculation on my fingers, I figured out that I'd been out cold for over three hours. I also discovered I had a drain under my left arm, meaning that more than the sentinel lymph nodes had been removed - an axial excision, not good news on the pathology-report front, and the five-day radiation protocol was off the table - which in turn meant I'd be a guest in the hospital overnight. Axial excision meant I had a Jackson-Pratt drain in my left armpit, which called for me to be "monitored"overnight.

Oh, joy.

I was rolled upstairs to a room – a private one, by luck alone – and the nurses, my sister, and my Terminator hovered around asking if I wanted anything.

Yes, I'd like lunch, please. I haven't eaten since yesterday.

There was some to-ing and fro-ing about where the nearest Panera Bread was – soup and sandwich was what I craved – and during that discussion I made a discovery. My left boob, which was now stitched and bandaged, was swollen. Not only was it swollen, it was swelling. It looked like Mt. St. Helen's just before it blew its stack, with blood playing the part of lava.

Hurried consultation with Dr. Sure Hands' husband-the-surgical-oncologist, who happened to be on the floor at the time, led to the conclusion that I needed to get back to the OR, stat. Off I rolled.

I woke up from anesthesia for the second time that day with surgeons still working on me. Couldn't feel a thing, but I was awake. They were talking about one of my favorite subjects, scuba diving, so I joined the discussion. They managed to contain their surprise, buttoned me up, and then rolled me back upstairs.

Apparently, a tiny artery had been nicked during the lumpectomy. It was small enough that it wasn't noticed at the time, but after an hour or so it got tired of being ignored and blew its top. Lucky me – two trips to the OR in one day. Do I know how to live, or what?

Things will not go as planned. Plan on it. That works for all parts of life, and seems particularly prevalent in health care.

Cancer For Christmas

I finally got my soup and sandwich at around 7pm. After we ate, my crew left, and I watched "Prison Break", thinking about busting out of the hospital.

I worked on trying to sleep, drifting off around midnight. I woke up around 2:30, with an aching left boob. I rang for the nurse, and asked over the intercom for some Vicodin, which I'd been taking since I returned the second time from the OR. A nurse with a Romanian accent said she'd be right in with the morphine.

No, I said, I don't need morphine. Vicodin would be just fine. Vlad the Nurse came in within seconds, holding a syringe, which contents she jammed into my IV. She said that would make me feel much better, and left.

It didn't make me feel better. Within seconds, I felt like I was on fire, with ants running through my bloodstream. I clutched the call button, figuring that I'd mash it hard if I felt my airway closing up. Luckily, that didn't happen, and after about twenty minutes the fire and ants subsided. I made a mental note for myself: self, it appears you're allergic to morphine. Remember to check that off on any future medical questionnaires.

I managed to survive the night without any further input from Vlad, or any other, nurses. The next morning, after a quick visit from Dr. Sure Hands, I was discharged - and allowed to walk to the waiting car. No wheelchair. Maybe I'd turned the corner, and it would all be A-OK from here.

Under the heading of Strange Discoveries Made Under Even Stranger Circumstances, here's a little factoid that I'm sure you'll find useful: if you find yourself with a surgery site that you can't get wet, and a deep desire for a shower, here's the fix – Glad Press-n-Seal. I kid you not – it sticks to your skin around the bandage, and allows you to shower, even wash your hair, as long as you keep the bandaged/Press-n-Sealed area out of direct contact with the shower spray.

Since I had a drain under my arm, and a large bandage over it, and over the surgery site on my breast, that I couldn't get wet, this was a great tip. One that let me shower the day after surgery, and feel almost human. Human with a few chunks missing, but human.

Dr. Sure Hands taught me that. I told you she was good, didn't I?

I got the full pathology report a week later, on Jan. 22, 2008:

Invasive ductal carcinoma

1.3 X 0.7 X 0.6cm tumor (not too big)

clean margins (they got it all)

0-3 lymph node positive (21 nodes taken, 1 dirty/20 clean)

no vascular invasion (hadn't entered my bloodstream)

Cancer For Christmas

HER-2/neu negative (this is good news – HER-2 positive means treatment with herceptin, which can have serious cardio-pulmonary side effects)

Progesterone positive (more good news – very effective treatment available to prevent recurrence of hormone-positive breast cancer)

Estrogen positive (see above)

High proliferation rate (sucker was growing fast, good thing I got my mammogram)

What all this added up to was Stage IIa - not terrible, and if it hadn't been detected in my annual mammogram, it would have gotten worse quickly due to that high proliferation rate.

That one dirty lymph node gave me the strong feeling that prudence dictated at least some sort of chemotherapy. I was not, however, terribly excited about wearing my cancer diagnosis on my head. I was still trying to get a consulting practice off the ground, and my gold-standard goal was retainer clients. I didn't want a potential customer to wonder if the retainer time frame would outlast my life expectancy.

The wig-and-hat play wouldn't fly, since I've always been the first one on my block to break out in a sweat as soon as the temperature goes over 75. That old aphorism that "horses sweat, men perspire, and ladies glisten" always makes me want to whinny. If I put on a hat, unless I'm outdoors in the winter, I wind up sweating like Dick Cheney at an anger management seminar. The few times I donned a wig back in my days as a wannabe actress told me that wigs were worse than hats – they made me sweat like Albert Brooks in "Broadcast News".

Ergo, I wanted to know if it was absolutely necessary for me to lose my hair to chemotherapy.

Meanwhile, my surgery scars had healed so well that the only way anyone would even notice I had any would be if I got held up on a nude beach – when I hold my hands up over my head, the missing chunk is visible. Arms down, invisible.

Dr. Sure Hands is damn good.

The Gift

Learn everything you can, make your choices based on that knowledge, and then surrender to the process. Plan, and then trust. And be prepared for the unexpected!

Chapter 6

THEN THEY POISON YOU
(PASS THE PICKLES, PLEASE)

I presented myself on a rainy Friday morning in early February at the office of Dr. Cocktail, an oncologist who had been recommended by Dr. Sure Hands. Another woman, making me two-for-two on female doctors since my diagnosis. Dr. Sure Hands had, I'm certain, referred me to her because she'd endured the grilling I was giving doctors, and knew that Dr. Cocktail would be equal to the challenge.

Right away, I knew I was in the right place. Dr. Cocktail had a sense of humor, laughing when she told me it was not at all a requirement that I lose my hair to chemotherapy. She offered to show me how different treatments stacked up, using a web-based tool for oncologists.

I'd been looking at that very website, AdjuvantOnline. com, and had seen the tools available for calculating the impact of a variety of treatment approaches on long-term cancer survivability. I'd seen the tools, but hadn't been able to use them, since I didn't have the secret handshake - a login and password, available only to registered medical professionals.

Here was my chance: a real doctor, with a real computer.

Dr. Cocktail said that six treatments with an older-line drug, CMF (cytoxan, methotrexate, and 5-fluorouracil), which had been the gold standard for breast cancer before anthracylines and taxols hit the scene, would, along with the lumpectomy, radiation, and hormone suppression drugs, put me around 90% on the 10 year survivability scale, while only thinning my hair a bit. Since I could be a hair donor, this didn't sound like a problem, and 90% put me in the A-/B+ range, which was my grade average throughout my school career.

I figured I'd stick with my historical average. CMF, here I come.

I found out later that afternoon that a good friend of mine, Patricia, who survived Stage IV breast cancer in the mid-1990s, had been treated with CMF. She told me that Dr. Cocktail hadn't lied about the not-losing-your-hair part, that it had taken ten months of treatments to make her a cue-ball. I'd only be on it for four months.

Patricia had been on CMF for 12 months. She has a lovely collection of wigs that her husband won't let her get rid of – I believe I've heard him mention them in the same sentence with "playtime," but I didn't pursue the subject. Not my playground!

Cancer For Christmas

The current gold standards for breast cancer, AC (anthracycline and cytoxan) or AT (anthracycline and taxol), pretty much guarantee that during the weeks between treatments 1 and 2, your hair will come out in clumps, bringing you that cue-ball-bald cancer badge.

Bottom line on chemotherapy, in my opinion, is that all chemo is crafted and targeted to fight Stage IV, with earlier stage patients just getting fewer treatments. The current gold standard for whatever you've got – breast cancer, lung cancer, lymphoma, whatever – might be the way to go, but you should ask what side effects to expect, what this particular treatment protocol will do to increase your long-term survival, and what other treatments might be available that could be as effective.

It's your body, it's your treatment, make sure you're part of the decision-making process.

Stay INSIDE the car when you're going through the car-wash.

BLOG POST 2/1/08

Catchin' the Chemo Bus
Well, I now know what the next seven (!) months of my life will look like. Luckily, all seven months won't be chemo (oy – what a thought!), but almost five will, starting on Feb. 11 and ending (it appears) on May 27. I'll get June "off", and then have radiation treatments July through August.

The decision on chemo was left up to me, and after lots of research and some statistical modeling, I discovered that a treatment protocol that included chemo, radiation, and 5 years of hormone suppression drugs puts me in the 90% zone for "still cancer-free in 10 years". That's an A-/B+, and since I was all about the grades in school, I'll stick with that approach here!

The good news? The chemo they're going to give me is not the bald-and-barfing variety. I won't feel great, but I won't feel dead, and I won't be wearing my cancer diagnosis on my head. That IS indeed good news, trust me.

The financial impact of this lovely dance I find myself doing is still revealing itself. Medical insurance is da bom, and I do have some, but the co-pays on my current plan are hideous. My insurance – my almost-former husband's company plan, that I developed – was decided on in '05, when I was on no meds, stayed healthy by working out and eating right, and was celebrating a 50 lb. weight loss. Believe me, I wish I'd had a way to see into the future!

Enough people have asked if they can "help", including someone who has offered to administer a trust if I set one up, that I will be talking to First Market Bank on Monday about how to do just that. I'll keep you posted, and if you'd like to help me with treatment costs...that will be how.

The best help, though, is really just continued good karma – I am still utterly convinced that I'll get through this 110% fine. And, boy, will I have some great stories at the end of this...!

———————

Infusion chemotherapy is typically delivered via either a PICC (peripherally inserted central catheter) line tied into a vein in your arm, or a TIVAS (totally implantable venous access system) called a portacath under the skin in your upper chest, fed into the subclavian vein under your clavicle.

Since I'd lost 21 lymph nodes to an axial excision, the PICC line wasn't an option – my left arm can no longer even have a blood pressure cuff on it, or blood drawn from it, and I'm also at risk for lymphedema, a chronic swelling of the arm due to lymphatic congestion. If your lymph system can't drain properly, the fluid backs up in the affected area. You also have a higher risk of infection if you get a wound on an arm or leg that has lymphedema. Add to that the risk that a PICC line would likely blow out the vein it was tied to in my right arm, making blood draws almost impossible in the future – not a good idea.

I had the portacath installed by Dr. Sure Hands on Feb. 8. Over the next few months I took to calling it my buzzer. Hit the buzzer, win a prize. Actually, I'd win the prize, which was getting to cancer-free. A portacath allows drug delivery and blood draws with an absolute minimum of fuss – good oncology nurses can hook you up in seconds, after a nice little 'freeze', where they hit you with a freeze spray to deaden the nerves in your skin just before they jack you into the Matr...um, attach you to the infusion machine.

I started chemo on Monday, Feb. 11. An additional mitzvah from Dr. Cocktail came that morning, when I told her I hadn't slept through the night since Dec. 10, and that first funky mammogram. She said, "We can fix that," and wrote me a scrip for Ambien. I used it for the next two weeks, and it worked like a charm. In fact, it still does. Don't have to take it every night, but a few nights a month it really comes in handy.

By now, you must realize that I'm someone who speaks up. In fact, most of my life, various ones have told me to pipe down, quit rocking the boat. When it's MY boat – my body, and what happens to it – I'll stop rocking it ten minutes after I'm dead. I encourage you to take the same tack.

Medical treatment really is a car-wash – they hook your wheels onto their conveyer belt, and off you go, getting washed, waxed, and whirly-towel-beaten to a fare-thee-well.

Why would you not ask questions, speak up, make your voice heard?

Doctors want to help – at least, most of them do. Some of them would make great prison guards, but that's a story for another day. The problem with medicine is that, in addition to being a calling, it's also a business.

Cancer For Christmas

That it's a business isn't the problem, the problem arises from how that business' operating model has changed over the last thirty years – thanks to 'managed care.'

I'll hold my thoughts on that for later.

Blog Post 2/16/2008

Oceans & Oceans of...Poison?

I had my first chemo treatment this last Monday, 2/11 (Happy Valentine's Day! Early!), and so far the after-effects have been weird, but manageable. I keep thinking of cartoons where some character starts quivering, and then his head explodes into a Dali-esque fright mask with, oh, a foot springing out of his forehead.

That hasn't happened. Yet.

What is happening is that instead of my usual eat-like-a-garbage-truck self, I've become someone who has to think hard about what might be edible. The data sheet on my chemo cocktail lists this side effect as "anorexia"– which makes me laugh so hard I can barely breathe. My name and anorexia in the same sentence? Get outta town.

The closest analogue I can come up with for the current eating sitch is this: back inna day, when I did offshore sailing, there were more than a few times that the rest of the crew was crawling around on the deck, beggin' to die. At those times, my experience was usually, "well,

I don't feel GREAT, but how about I make some soup?" The most memorable version of this was twenty years ago, delivering the schooner ORIANDA from Lauderdale to Tortola. The skipper decided to leave Lauderdale literally on the tail of a hurricane (luckily only a weakening Cat 1), just before midnight.

No, it didn't seem like a great idea to me, either, but a ship is not a democracy.

Another woman on the crew and I had drawn 12-4 watch, meaning we were first up, and would be fighting the Gulf Stream by 2am. When we did hit the Stream, we had 15-foot cross-seas and were shipping green water over both bows. My watch-partner and I were literally tied to the boat (as one always should be offshore), taking turns steering, which was like trying to wrestle an anaconda. At about 3am, the engine started to sputter – the skipper and the mechanic headed into the engine room to see whassup. Diagnosis: busted fuel hose.

The engine room was off the pilothouse, which was directly in front of the steering station. In order to work on the engine, the pilothouse light needed to be on. In order to see the compass and steer a course, the helmsman needed to have the pilothouse light OFF. We struck a compromise – I would hold the pilothouse hatch doors closed and shield them with my body, preventing the light from hitting the helmsman in the face and thereby risking a course change for Havana. Or Maine.

So, there I was, holding the hatch doors closed as heavy

diesel fumes rolled past, and the boat tossed around like we were driving through a washing machine on full agitate.

For the first time in my sailing life, I felt seasick.

What I wanted most right then – other than for things to settle down, just a bit, or for blessed dawn to break – was some coffee. And some soup. Which I got, a few hours later, once the dawn did break and I could get down to the galley (I was ship's cook), clear away the debris from the rough passage, and get things going.

So, chemo "anorexia" for me is being seasick, or like eating like a 10-year-old. PB&J sandwiches, mac-n-cheese with grilled chicken, chicken noodle soup. My usual chili, garlic, and stinky cheese palate has vanished. It's only until June, though – who knows, maybe I'll feel better about bathing suit season after this.

The above anecdote tells the story of my chemo experience pretty well. I had a much better ride than I had thought I would, much easier than other people I shared the infusion room with during those months that I reported for ritual poisoning every third Monday.

The most memorable thing that happened during my chemo treatment was only parenthetically related to treatment – it was the departure of Dr. Cocktail from the practice, one week after my first treatment, which left me in the hands of the man I came to call Dr. Drive-by.

Remember Dr. Surgeon Ego? Dr. Drive-by was his oncology/hematology peer – on the surface, very friendly, with what I'm sure he thought of as great bedside manner and a very caring persona.

Um, no.

Over the following few months, I had an opportunity to thank my lucky stars that I hadn't developed my treatment plan with him. He was, after all, the doctor. He knew what you were supposed to do, and he was going to tell you what that was. Then you were going to do it.

Questions? Maybe you got an answer, but you had to listen fast. He was in and out of the exam room so fast I'd find myself thinking, "did he say something? I don't think he did, did he?"

Every visit was a drive-by with Dr. Drive-by.

Another thing about him that had me wondering why he'd chosen medicine, particularly oncology, as a profession was the fact that his cologne hit the room before he did. I'd swear he marinated himself in the stuff. Think about it: you're undergoing chemotherapy treatment, your nose and your stomach have become hypersensitive, you get nauseated easily...and here comes some dude marinated in Polo Ralph Lauren? It's enough to gag a maggot, trust me.

I missed Dr. Cocktail, but the oncology nurses at this practice were outstanding– I stayed because of them, particularly Crystal and Faith. They were flesh and blood angels. They always had the most tender touch, and I'll remember them with love for the rest of my days.

Also, the practice had required that Dr. Cocktail sign a six-month non-compete, meaning that she wouldn't be back on the radar until sometime in August. So, I was stuck with Dr. Drive-by, and the angels of the infusion room.

Those wonderful women were the ones who really took care of me. He just signed the forms.

There were some bright spots during this phase of treatment:

BLOG POST 2/20/08

Punch-lines I Resist with Supreme Effort, Part 1
OK, I realize that Valentine's Day was last week. Call me slow, put me on the short bus, and let's move on.

I got yet another weird gift (remember "Cancer for Christmas"?), this time in service of my chemo-blasted palate. A friend who survived Stage IV breast cancer in 1994 was on the same chemo cocktail they've got me on, and recommended dill pickles as the fix for chemo-metal-mouth, the metallic taste that chemo leaves behind as it poisons the **** outta your entire system.

I shared that data with a number of friends, including the one with whom I have the most complicated relationship. In a nutshell, we have a vibrant friendship that includes pretty much every feature of a long-term relationship: agreement, disagreement, laughter, companionable silence, ridiculous adventures, mutual discoveries...everything except sex. Which, after 10 years without, I'm really wishing would reappear at some point.

Considering that 10 year drought includes a 7-year marriage (how ****ing sad is THAT?), to say I feel ripe for the plucking would be a vast understatement.

ANYway, I shared the planned pickle ploy. On 2/14, I got an email asking me if I had a drecky taste in my mouth. I did. He then asked if FedEx had arrived yet. It hadn't, and he replied a bit later that whatever-it-was apparently wouldn't arrive until the next day, 2/15.

FedEx, on 2/15, delivered...a Pickle Palooza. From The Pickle Guys on Essex St. on the Lower East Side (NYC), the purveyors of my pickle preference for all the years I lived in NY.

He had me at half-sour.

Cancer For Christmas

Keep your pedestrian Valentine's Day chocolate. I'm all about the pickle.

_____

Then there were the scary moments.

When I reported for my third chemo treatment, the lab report on my blood levels had some warning signs – my neutrophils, the bacteria-fighting part of my white blood cells, were dangerously low. Normal is 2.0-6.9 k/uL (2000-6900 per cubic millimeter, or mm3). Mine was down at .8, or 800 mm3.

Dr. Drive-by, in his fast dance through the exam room, said that most doctors won't treat patients below 1000 mm3, but he would, and to call him if I got a fever.

At the time of that conversation, I had no idea what a neutrophil even was. I had my treatment, and then dashed home to consult Dr. Google.

Neutrophil: Specific type of white blood cell; plays a role in fighting infections.

Further reading scared the crap outta me. At levels below 1000 mm3, infection risk goes up about 20%. Once it gets to 500 mm3, naturally occurring bacteria in your body, like the e. coli that swarm in everyone's gut, can cause an infection. Oh, boy, just what I need – 10 days in the hospital hooked up to an antibiotic IV. I was at 800 mm3, and all Dr. Drive-by had for me was "call me if you get a fever"??

I was determined not to wind up in the hospital. I had enough challenges already.

My reading and research (notes on this are in the Resources & References chapter at the end of the book) all seemed to agree on one point: don't eat any raw food. For a salad freak like me, this was a real problem – my fridge is usually full of lettuce, celery, scallions, tomatoes, greens, and other fresh produce, which I blend together into salads and meals of all kinds.

I put all the salad stuff in grocery bags and took it over to a friend's house, and told her that she'd won the salad lottery.

Further reading indicated that red and orange fruits and vegetables were great neutrophil boosters: beets, cantaloupe, tomatoes, carrots, mangoes, and sweet potatoes are all high in beta carotene, which helps boost the immune system. Cantaloupe and mangoes I could eat raw, since their skins are removed before you scarf 'em up.

Beets, carrots, and sweet potatoes were all skinned before cooking, and tomatoes were always cooked, too.

Dark green vegetables like spinach, broccoli, kale, and chard are beta carotene treasure troves as well, and all taste great steamed. I also discovered that shitake mushrooms have an immunity builder called lentinan in them, and that beef and other red meats are high in zinc, another powerful immune booster. Add garlic, my ultimate favorite food on the planet, and you've got a smokin' good grocery list.

I started living on a diet of steak, sautéed mushrooms, roasted red peppers, broiled tomatoes, and sweet potatoes, with steamed broccoli and greens, mangoes, and cantaloupe singing backup. All of this – well, not the cantaloupe, but everything else – had plenty of garlic on it. Since all of these are on my favorite-foods list, life was looking pretty sweet.

I was pissed beyond belief that Dr. Drive-by hadn't bothered to share any information with me about neutropenia, which is the official medical term for a low neutrophil count. I was further prodded toward sputtering rage by the fact that, when I called to ask him if I could be treated with a netrophil-boosting drug like Neulasta before treatment #4, he said, "no." No explanation, just "no."

I kept up with my red/orange plant, red meat, garlic, and mushroom regimen, and when I reported for treatment #4, my neutrophil count had gone from 800 mm3 to 1400 mm3 – a 57% increase.

Of course, now Dr. Drive-by was all about the $2,000 shot (that's the cost of one dose of Neulasta, and no, I'm NOT kidding), and he pooh-poohed my idea that I'd boosted my neutrophil count through diet.

So I appeared the next day for my Neulasta blast. I'm not a wimp, but that shot hurts like hell. And the aftermath includes bone pain, because what the drug is doing is hammering your bone marrow to pump out more neutrophils. My hip joints felt like rusty hinges for a week afterward.

The oncology nurses asked me about my dietary approach, and I told them, asking them to share the info with any patients who wanted to do some immune-boosting on their own during treatment. It's a healthy diet, whether you're a chemo patient or just looking to avoid getting a cold. I'm still on it, even though chemo ended months ago.

BLOG POST 3/26/08

Dispatch From Cancer Camp

It's been a while – time to bring you up to date on all the fun we're having here at Cancer Camp!

I have to say that the counselors here are very strange – they've all got knives and other sharp pointy objects they just can't stop poking me with. Also, the activities suck, since they mostly involve sitting around getting poisoned. I have been advised that coming up on my activities list is the exciting "burn Casey's left side to a crisp" game, a/k/a radiation treatment. Wow, that sure sounds like fun, don't it?

Actually, things have been surprisingly low-stress,

considering that it's now been over three months that my name and the word cancer have been included in the same sentence. I truly feel that I've got this lovely visit from the Cancer Troll beat, and once I get past all the 'treatment', I'll never see the Troll again.

This past Monday marked the mid-point of ritual poisoning (chemo – three down, three to go), and in addition to the anorexia - still makes me laugh, sayin' that about myself - I spoke of in my last dispatch, I've discovered the joys of chemo-brain. I didn't notice it after the first round of chemo, likely because I was so concerned with what the physical effects would be that I didn't expect much of myself that first week. Since the effects seemed so manageable, after the second chemo session I thought I'd just keep on keepin' on.

Um, no. Not really.

I couldn't write a freakin' press release that week. I TEACH people how to write press releases. I had all the details for a media advisory about an event for an organization I work with here, I had promised them I'd have it to them by that Friday...and I could not, for the life of me, figure out where to begin. Not on Wednesday, not on Thursday, not on Friday. Couldn't get my **** together, mentally, until Sunday, and even then it was an effort. Totally on the short bus, all that week.

So this week I'm moving slowly, expecting not much from myself, and warning all that my output might be, um, minimal. And sleeping like you would not believe

– ten hours at a stretch, with short sinking spells in the afternoon. The cure isn't quite worse than the disease… however, it's still not something I'd recommend as a "must" on one's life list!

Business for Mighty Casey Media seems to be developing – at last! – and it appears that 2008 might just be my year, as I had set forth in my first-ever annual plan, drawn up just before the Troll appeared. The Casey Kicks Cancer Trust is helping with my medical care costs, and some basic expenses (rent & utilities) as I work to get MCM to the point that it's actually supporting me.

The generosity of friends has been remarkable, including a trio of women who gave me an iPod Nano (an EIGHT GIG iPod Nano!) just before my 2nd round of chemo, which saved me from the truly horrible fate of listening to commercial radio in the infusion room. There's enough room on this thing for my entire CD collection (which is over 600 at this point), with space still left for more. I absolutely LOVE this thing!

So, thanks to all of you for your emotional and practical support – I'll update everyone again next month, and we'll have a big virtual celebration in late May, when chemo's over!

BLOG POST 3/30/08

Beeting Up On Myself

As a person participating in the fun-filled romp known as chemotherapy, your 'umble correspondent has been able to make all sorts of wonderful discoveries.

Cancer For Christmas

There was "anorexia", wherein our heroine was introduced to the practice of picky eating. Not something she had been familiar with previously, at all.

There was "chemo-brain", wherein she learned just how stupid "dumber than a box of rocks" really was. Is. Whatever.

Today, she learned that the two can be combined in new and interesting ways.

Say, f'rinstance, one learns that one's blood is dangerously low in something called neutrophils - due to the aforementioned chemotherapy's Sherman-like march through one's bloodstream toward whatever cancer cells might have the temerity to remain within one's corpus. (Note: there ain't none, one just has to run the bases, like any other home-run hitter.)

One reads up on neutrophils, and white blood counts, learning that a diet rich in beef, cooked mushrooms, and red/orange/yellow vegetables is just the ticket for getting that neutrophil level back up to the mark that will prevent our heroine from getting hit with Neulasta. That being the drug used to hammer one's marrow into manufacturing neutrophils, while also apparently causing bone pain - IOW, not something our heroine is inclined to entertain the deployment of, since she's got entirely enough chemicals runnin' 'round her veins, thank you very MUCH.

Anywise, the thought of some yummy beets seems like a good thing, and she hits the local Kroger in search thereof. What ho! Organic beets! With greens on top! On Wednesday, the beets are steamed and enjoyed, with a steak and sautéed 'shrooms. Yum. She feels better already.

The greens were left in the veg crisper, and today's lunchtime seemed like just the time to wilt 'em, butter/salt 'em, and get outside 'em. So she did.

Oh - has it been mentioned that a regular side effect of chemo involves the, um, acceleration of elimination of the alimentary sort?

We think she set some kind of land speed record around the time from beet-green ingestion to beet-green removal. The old aphorism about what goes fast through a goose came to mind.

Beet feet, indeed.

The things one can learn when one isn't paying attention....

My chemo experience became predictable, which made life a little easier to manage. I knew to expect chemo-brain during the first week, as well as what I called the 'icks'. Both were manageable: the first by managing expectations, both my own and my clients'; the second with anti-nausea medication.

The second week, I'd start feeling pretty good, and the third week I'd feel positively terrific. Then it was back for my ritual poisoning, my visit with Dr. Drive-by, and ministrations from the infusion-room goddesses.

I had a Neulasta treatment on April 15, and again on May 6. I tried to wave off the second Neulasta hit, since my neutrophil count was back up in the normal range by then. Dr. Drive-by's response? He threatened to delay my next treatment if I didn't submit to the second Neulasta shot. No real explanation, just, "do you want to delay your next treatment? If not, you're getting Neulasta."

Prince of a guy, that Dr. Drive-by.

My last chemo infusion was on Thursday, May 22 – I asked to move up the date, since the third Monday would have been Memorial Day, and I wanted to get this phase of my life over with as soon as possible. Do you blame me? I was due back in the office on Friday, May 23 for my Neulasta treatment. Did I go? What do you think?

Hell, no. I was done. And I didn't think it was worth $2,000, anyway.

My last interaction with Dr. Drive-by was in the infusion room, during my last treatment. He swanned in, sat on a small rolling stool and rolled over to sit before me. He was clutching a small paper bag. He looked deep into my eyes, and said, "these are for you. The instructions are clear, but call me if you have any questions."

I thanked him, and he rolled/swanned back out. I looked in the bag, and saw a 28-day supply of Arimidex, one of the aromitase inhibitor drugs used to treat hormone positive breast cancer in post-menopausal women.

He might not listen to his patients much, but he does great work for Astra Zeneca.

Blog post (5/23/2008)

Off the Chemo Bus

Yesterday marked the end of my trip down Poison Lane, a/k/a chemo. To say that I'm glad to see the Chemo Bus pull away, leaving me at the curb, would be another in a series of vast understatements.

I learned all sorts of things during my bus ride, including:
There are doctors who don't tell you much, even if you ask lots of questions.

Nurses are da bom, particularly oncology nurses.

A patient must be her own advocate, even if her doctor is communicative, because a doctor will only answer the questions you ask.

Cancer For Christmas

Never, ever, eat beet greens all by themselves, particularly if it's one's first meal of the day...!

Blog Post 5/26/08

OK, so now I'm back to the lovely surgery center tomorrow. Why am I flashing on Hilly-the-Sheltie just post-tooth-pull, coming out of anesthesia, with her tongue hanging out of slack jaws and what really looked like little Xs in her eyes? I guess that's what one looks like coming 'round, but what a prospect! 'Specially since a friend is picking me up...

It's been an interesting trip through the medical car-wash so far. My relentless research and informed inquiry has allowed me to sit inside the car – not asking questions, not making sure your voice is present in treatment planning, can mean that you get strapped to the hood, getting whapped by the spinning towel things and lots of soap & wax up your nose.

I've had a very easy ride, only feeling icky a few days out of every treatment cycle. The meds have taken good care of those icks, and other than those few days, the only effect I've felt is that I tire more easily than I used to – I've been able to exercise, carry on with (what might pass for) working to build my business, putting one foot in front of the other pretty much every day.

I do believe I figured out the very best outcome of this particular pass – I'm writing a book, "Cancer for Christmas", that will detail my time at Cancer Camp.

Books by cancer survivors tend to be more about spiritual uplift and positive attitude. Attitude I've got in spades, but what I want to share is the research I did; what my approach was; the tools I found most useful; how to be an active participant in your treatment and recovery.

I won't be able to finish C4C until I have my next mammogram and/or MRI in December. I hope to have it out in early '09. Watch this space.

Next step in treatment is scheduled to be radiation. If I acquiesce to getting burnt to a crisp, that will be over in early August. Then it's five years of aromitase inhibitors (in civilian-speak: hormone suppression drugs), which will be the last brick in the wall between me and any more visits from the Cancer Troll.

I headed over to Dr. Sure Hands' office on Tuesday, May 27 for removal of my portacath, and some scar revision on that wounded warrior, my left breast.

It had been 158 days since I got my strange Christmas present. I had managed to keep a roof over my head, and my bills paid, with the support of family, friends, customers, and even people I didn't know, through the Casey Kicks Cancer Trust.

I belong to a Curves gym, and the owner of the club where I am a member had worked with the managers of her three clubs on a fundraiser for the Trust. Each club made t-shirts with their club name, and a graphic. My club, Curves Short Pump in the western suburbs of Richmond, VA, designed theirs with a cheetah print. I wear mine with pride, and deep gratitude.

I had now survived diagnosis, surgery, and chemo, I still faced radiation treatment, which was due to start in late June.

The Gift

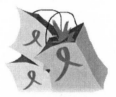

Oncology nurses, who can help you overlook some really bad doctor behavior. And real pickles. And the overwhelming gift of support from friends.

Chapter 7

THEN THEY BURN YOU
(HIROSHIMA, MON AMOUR)

Radiation treatment is lumped in with lumpectomy.

When you're talking to your doctor(s) about treatment, it seems like it's one long word: lumpectomy-and-radiation. I'd spent lots of time talking with Dr. Sure Hands before surgery. I'd spent a good bit of time with Dr. Cocktail before embarking on chemotherapy. I'd had a meeting on Feb. 12 with Dr. Glow Worm, the radiation oncologist that every breast cancer survivor I knew had recommended highly.

She (hey, I'm stickin' with the girls, remember?) had given me an outline of treatment, and told me to schedule a planning session after I'd finished chemo. We did that on June 12, and I started treatment on June 24.

I had hoped to get radiation over with by the end of July. Unfortunately, Dr. Glow Worm had other plans – she prescribed 35 treatments, which meant seven weeks of once-a-day radiation hits, Monday through Friday.

Cancer For Christmas

Since radiation had seemed to be no big deal, just the second part of that compound word, lumpectomy-and-radiation, I figured I'd breeze through it. I'd read and heard that it made you tired, but hey, I'd survived almost four months of chemo – how could radiation be anything but a breeze after that?

Wrong again, Spanky.

Radiation was a massive serving of tired, with a side order of burnt-to-a-crisp. The first two weeks weren't too bad, with a worsening burn the only apparent problem. By the middle of the third week, though, I felt 80 years old, and my poor left boob looked, and felt, like a burrito that had been left in the microwave on high for a week.

Stiff, lumpy, and burnt.

I also developed a full-blown case of lymphedema.

As pissed off as I had been at Dr. Drive-by, I hadn't bothered to get in his face about my issues with him. It didn't seem worth it, since he had that 'I'm the doctor" thing going on, and that can be pretty impenetrable.

Dr. Glow Worm didn't get a pass. She had talked about the possibility of swelling during our initial sessions, but had never said the word lymphedema. If she had, I would have fastened on to that, and we would have had a deeper discussion.

When I looked in the mirror one morning, and realized that my upper left arm and elbow were noticeably larger than the right, I got scared, and then I got mad.

My late mother-in-law battled breast cancer in the '60s, back in the bad old days when radical mastectomy was the only treatment option offered by surgeons. Her entire left side had essentially been ripped off, and she had developed lymphedema quickly after surgery. Her left arm was swollen to about four times the size of the right – her grandson, my step-son, had referred to it as her 'Popeye arm' when he was a small child. Her condition was permanent, because it had never been treated. She'd been told it was just part of what happened to breast cancer patients.

I knew what lymphedema was, I knew that I was at risk, and now I had it. I was angry that it seemed that radiation had brought it on, but that I hadn't been told about that possibility.

There's a big difference between the words 'swelling' and 'lymphedema'.

I got up in Dr. Glow Worm's grill about this. Her response was that I needed to see a shrink because I, and I quote, "clearly have issues."

I'll admit to 'issues' – I'm convinced that most of those issues are caused by poor communication. Sometimes that fault can certainly be mine, but in this instance I felt that it was clearly hers, her failure to communicate fully with me that radiation can bring on lymphedema, not just "swelling".

This really challenged my "leave the Samsonite behind" epiphany, too – was I losing my grip on letting go? Yes, I know, I can't help it, puns just happen around me. Seriously, though, I thought long and hard about why this made me so damned mad – there was a bit of fear and frustration in there, but I really did feel as though I hadn't been clearly and fully informed.

The question now was: what do I do about it?

Back in the days when my mother-in-law was dealing with the aftermath of breast cancer surgery, there wasn't much that she could do. There wasn't much for a doctor to do, either. In the last couple of decades, the pioneers in lymphedema treatment have all been European. Slowly, the medical establishment in the U.S. has recognized that early treatment with manual lymphatic drainage (MLD) massage, exercise, and well-fitted compression garments is the best approach to controlling and managing lymphedema. Lymphedema clinics are appearing in many medical centers.

Lucky for me that one of those lymphedema clinics is within a few miles of my house, isn't it?

In addition to the suggestion that I see a shrink (no, thanks, I'll hang on to my righteous rage), Dr. Glow

Worm also gave me a referral to the lymphedema clinic at St. Mary's Hospital here in Richmond.

If you've got lymphedema, these are just the girls you want to hang out with – not only are they outstanding masseuses, they're highly trained medical professionals who really understand their specialty. They helped me get some lovely custom-made compression sleeves that I wear fairly frequently, and always when I fly.

I love it that I have a medical excuse to book a massage.

I'll deal with lymphedema – my breast cancer souvenir - for the rest of my life. The swelling in my left arm has lessened somewhat, and I have heard from many other lymphedema patients that around six months after radiation treatment ends, lymphedema in the affected arm can be minimal. It's been almost five months as I write this, and I am seeing improvement.

But it will never go away completely.

Radiation treatment continued until Aug. 8, two days after my 56th birthday. Happy birthday to me. From early July through August, I was so tired I could barely think. I could focus on project work for up to three hours a day, the rest of the day I was essentially a potted plant.

If I had to do all this over again, I'd give some serious consideration to a mastectomy – mostly because it would mean I could avoid radiation treatment. That's how sick, and tired, it made me. I know it sounds extreme, but mastectomy with reconstruction is an option that I'd encourage anyone facing breast cancer to at least consider.

Giving yourself a chance to avoid getting nuked back to the Stone Age deserves some thought.

The Gift

Learning how to manage,
and deploy, anger in a way
that doesn't have blowback .

Chapter 8
THE DOCTOR IS IN

Richmond might call itself a city, but it's really a small town. In the months since Dr. Cocktail had fallen off the radar due to the non-compete with her former practice, I'd had my personal version of the underground telegraph working to find out when she'd be back in action. Other patients of hers heard about this, and started contacting me, asking me to let them know what I found out.

Small dots and dashes started to come through in late spring, when a good friend told me that a member of her pottery class at a local arts center was one of the top gynecologic oncologists in Richmond. I asked her to ask him if he knew Dr. Cocktail, and the word came back that he did. Not only did he know her, but she was talking about opening a practice in the same building where he worked his version of chemical magic.

I asked, again through the pottery phone, if he'd be willing to give her a letter from me. Reply: yes.

I wrote her a short note, saying I was looking forward to seeing her again to talk about follow-up treatment with hormone suppression drugs, and that I wasn't going to start taking the Arimidex that Dr. Drive-by had given me until she and I had re-connected.

The rest of the summer passed. I made it through the Bataan Death March called radiation treatment, and spent most of August trying to recover from the experience.

In late August, I'd gotten enough information that I decided to take matters in hand and start a campaign to track down Dr. Cocktail myself. I called the hospital where Dr. Gyn-Onc Pottery Dude had his practice, and asked for Dr. Cocktail.

Huzzah - I was given the number to her office!

I did a quick calculation on my fingers – February to March, one. To April, two. May, three. June, four. July, five. August...yippee! Six month non-compete complete!

I called, and got voicemail saying that everyone was in a meeting, call this other number. I did, and asked the woman who answered if I could make an appointment with Dr. Cocktail. This was Thursday, Aug. 21, and I asked for the earliest appointment available. I was told that would be Monday, Aug. 24 at 9:00am.

Book it, baby.

When I showed up at Dr. Cocktail's new digs, it was obvious she hadn't been there long. No computers yet, and a minimum of office furnishings and décor. However, the doctor was in, and guess what? I was her very first appointment in her new practice.

How cool was that?

I had done a lot of reading in the intervening months about aromitase inhibitors (AIs), and was well-versed in their side effects. In 20% of patients, they can bring on osteoporosis, and make any existing arthritis excruciatingly worse. I'd spoken to women who had been on an AI, and had had to stop taking it because their pain essentially immobilized them.

Dr. Cocktail and I both wanted to know what my bone-density starting point was – she said that her usual protocol was to put patients on Fosamax at the same time she prescribed an AI. I had a bone scan, and we waited for the results.

Both my parents had osteoporosis. My mother had had a tumor on her pituitary gland that was discovered when she was in her late 50s. Surgical removal of the gland was the only treatment option, which meant that she'd spent the rest of her life – 23 years – on cortico-steroids, which had caused osteoporosis. My father battled Parkinson's disease for 17 years, taking a vast cocktail of drugs which, along with the restriction on exercise caused by Parkinson's dyskenesia, brought on his osteoporosis.

Cancer For Christmas

I wasn't going to take any chances. If I had to take my AIs with a Fosamax chaser, that was fine with me. I enjoy dancing, yoga, the gym, biking, and activity in general too much to risk osteoporosis.

A few days later, Dr. Cocktail called with the results. After my ten month slog through the cancer treatment car-wash, I caught a huge break: my bone density was so good that Fosamax wasn't necessary. I could just keep doing whatever it was I was doing – which was regular weight-bearing exercise, healthy dairy products in my diet, and calcium citrate supplements – and start taking the AIs.

So I did. And, so far, the arthritis in my knees still hurts, but no worse than it did before I started taking Arimidex.

Yet another break. Let's see how many of those I can rack up!

Oh, and that letter that I'd given Dr. Gyn-Onc Pottery Dude? She'd gotten it...covered in clay.

The Gift

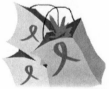

Learning to use indefatigability
(go look it up!) to get what you need,
when you need it, from the right person.

Chapter 9

BALLS DON'T MAKE YOU BRAVE, BUT TITS SURE CAN

Fall arrived. Life went on. Business continued to build, slow but steady. I felt pretty good.

It was time to book my annual mammogram.

I called the titanium-standard women's imaging center in town, the offices of Dr. ESDP. I had been meaning to check her out for a couple of years, and that resolve firmed up when I discovered that my beloved Dr. BD lacked the latest technology. He started with an analog X-ray film, which was converted to a digital image. Dr. ESDP's mammograms were all digital, all the way.

My appointment was scheduled for Tuesday, Dec. 23, 2008. 379 days since my 2007 mammogram, 369 days since I was diagnosed with breast cancer.

Time to cowgirl up.

I spent Thanksgiving in my hometown, Coronado CA, with my sister, my brother, his family, and a buffet of cousins, aunts, uncles, and life-long friends.

Cancer For Christmas

When I got home, I saw each day as a countdown to achieving true survivor status: M-day, 12/23/08. As that day drew closer, I kept thinking of that phrase 'whistling past the graveyard', and hoped that graveyard was far in the future.

I tried not to think about it. With no success at all. I went about all my daily routines, worked on projects for my clients, even worked on this book. But all if it happened with a rising level of pink noise in the background: M-day, 12/23/08.

Then, it arrived. M-day.

My appointment wasn't until 3:30pm, and I was reminded of Dec. 20, 2007, as I killed time until I could find out what the results of my biopsy were.

I had a busier day scheduled for M-day, with project work in the morning and a lunch with a potential customer scheduled for 11:30. After lunch, I wandered around town a bit, even hitting Wal-Mart two days before Christmas, which I admit proves I'm a masochist.

At 3:25, I walked through the door of Dr. ESDP's clinic, and checked in at the desk.

My medical insurance had terminated on Dec. 15, 2008. I had reason to be deeply grateful that hadn't happened in December 2007 – that would have made my journey almost impossibly difficult. When I was diagnosed with cancer, I had insurance that covered more than 90% of the costs (to date: approximately $120,000.00, meaning my direct costs so far have run around $10,000.00). That policy had not been renewed, because the monthly premiums would have been over $1,200.00 per month. My income can't support that level of expense in addition to the $5,000.00 deductible required by the policy.

I had joined the ranks of the uninsured.

Blog Post 12/15/2008

Pay No Attention to the Man Behind the Curtain
(If You'd Like to Stay Blissfully Ignorant)

I lost my health insurance the other day - and I'm not going to look for it.

I have reason to be very glad this didn't happen last year, given the cancer-for-Christmas gift I received at my mammogram last December.

Now that I'm in the self-pay column, I called the imaging practice where my next mammogram will take place to ask what the cost would be.

I have seen Explanation of Benefits (EOB) statements from my insurer - when I had one! - that listed the above-the-line cost as $600 to $1,000. Then there was the 'negotiated discount', and the other horse-trading hand signals that brought the cost down to around $350, which the insurer then paid the doctor.

Every EOB I've ever seen had this sort of dance on it - high initial cost, the insurer does a 'look what a great deal we got for you!' discount jig, and hey-presto, the final price is reduced by 50%-or-more.

So, when I called the imaging center, I was bracing myself for sticker shock.

I did get sticker shock, but in the other direction - a screening mammogram is $135, a diagnostic mammogram runs $120-$180, and ultrasound, if necessary, adds another $75.

Meaning the worst-case cost scenario is....$255.

Mention health care in any circle, and you'll hear cries about costs spiraling out of control, of doctors who lose money seeing HMO patients, of hospitals taking it in the shorts on equipment and supply costs, of patients paying $200 for an aspirin (I guess that's 'cause a nurse delivered it in a little paper cup?), of that last week of dad's life when his hospital bill hit $100K.

Here's a question - could it just be because of managed care that costs have managed to careen out of control? I'm old enough to remember that, back inna day, you went to the doctor and paid for your visit on the way out.

If you had a prescription, to went to the pharmacy and got it filled...and paid for it.

Needed lab work? You went to the lab, and paid the bill when it arrived.

You had insurance coverage against the day - which you hoped to avoid - when you'd have to go into the hospital.

Here's a suggestion for Tom Daschle, and the incoming Obama health care team: you don't need to invent a new system. Just go old-school, and add technology to it. Give consumers control not just over their care, but its cost.

When you're in the exam room with your doctor, thanks to managed care that's you, your doctor, and fifty people you can't see involved in decisions about your medical care.

That's fifty people who all want their 'taste', who add their cost - for administration, for oversight, for just taking up space in the transaction - to the cost of the actual visit.

That's the first way to attack cost - admit that the Great and Powerful Oz, the whole 'managed care' monolith, is really just a venal clerk behind a curtain who's inserted himself into the medical care system.

Putting doctors and their patients back in control of medical care - really - would not just help control costs, but it might also drive actual patient ownership of their health. Now there's an idea.

So here's a suggestion - kill managed care. And don't have a funeral.

That's my story, and I'm stickin' to it...

Surprised? I'm not. More on that later.

After I filled out the usual wad of forms, I was taken to a changing room where I be-gowned myself. I then retired to a room full of other be-gowned gals in some phase of their annual boob-squishing.

Then it was time for my annual boob-squishing. After what had happened after the last one, I was just a trifle nervous.

Actually, I was in the throes of slack-jawed terror.

The imaging tech was a sweet young woman who treated me like I deserved to have a good day. What a lovely thing that was.

She did her thing with a minimum of pain, which was an achievement since my wounded warrior left breast is still tender after all it's been through.

I then went back to the Waiting Room of the Be-gowned to await my results.

I'm a very fast reader. I think I went through three magazines while I waited, but my comprehension wasn't great. I wonder why.

Finally, a woman in a lab coat came to the door and said I could get dressed, and meet the doctor in her office at the end of the hall. I figured this was good news – they wouldn't tell me to get dressed if there was a problem, right?

I dressed, and went into the doctor's office. As I waited I paced back and forth, reading all of the degrees, citations, and thank-you letters on the wall. There were a lot of them.

The doctor came in, smiled, and said, "everything looks good. Come back in six months so we can keep an eye on the area around your scar tissue."

I burst into tears – well, I did my version of bursting into tears, which is I mist up a bit, and then I cowgirl up.

It doesn't take balls to be brave, it takes tits.

I celebrated my way out the door, posting a message on Twitter and Facebook that I was officially cancer-free. I headed over to a friend's place, a friend who is a 7-year survivor of Stage IV ovarian cancer. That's some surviving! We celebrated my official induction into the survivor's club with a glass of wine and some homemade fish chowder.

CaNceʳ Foʳ CHʳⁱStMₐS

After I left her place, I shared my news in a few other places, along with calls to family and friends to tell them the hard part of the journey was over. I'd gotten the best Christmas present of my life, two days early.

Blog Post 12/24/2008

Cancer for Christmas, One Year Later

I had my annual mammogram yesterday–remembering how last year's formerly routine event wound up, to say I was a little nervous is a vast understatement.

Here's the news: I'm now officially a survivor.

Looking back at the last 369 days, I have to say it's been quite a ride. So many people have helped me, have lifted me up, have kept me from feeling that terrible aloneness that's part of fighting a life-threatening disease.

'Thank you' sounds inadequate, but it comes from the deepest and most tender part of my heart.

I will finish the first draft of "Cancer for Christmas" by New Year's Day. Then it's on to finding an agent, a publisher, or – best of all possible worlds – both. I'll be reaching out to Save the Tatas and the Susan G. Komen Foundation, offering them a piece of the cover price in exchange for helping promote the book once it's published.

My goal is to help anyone in the fight – against cancer, or any other life-changing disease – navigate the medical car-wash and manage their medical care for their benefit.

Because if you don't, no one else will.

2008 has been quite a journey. I'm in an incredibly wonderful place, which I don't know that I would recognize had I not had my dance with the Cancer Troll.

2009 is already a mortal lock for my best year yet – I wish you the same!

The Gift

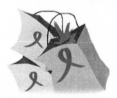

Survival is never guaranteed.
Keep asking for what you need,
keep pushing toward a win.
Odds are in your favor
if you just keep moving forward.

Chapter 10
WHAT I'VE LEARNED @ THE MEDICAL-CARE CAR-WASH

I've learned plenty in the last year – most of it falls into one of these categories:

Early detection is critical for cancer, or any other 'really big disease'

The medical community needs to revamp its 'I'm Parnassus, you're just the patient' culture

Medical insurers need to remove themselves from the doctor/patient relationship

All of us need to grow up, and take some meaningful actions to ensure our continuing health on an individual basis, every day

Let's take the lessons in order.

Early Detection Is Critical
Early detection is the #1 indicator of cancer survival. The earlier your cancer is found, the higher the likelihood that you'll be alive in 10 years.

Unfortunately, there are two things working against you:

Medicine is concentrating on finding a cure, with much less attention given to early detection. To be fair, cancer prevention gets a lot of attention, too, from 'quit smoking' to 'eat broccoli' public service announcements. Detection is still a distant third on where research money goes.

Here in the U.S., we've got a cultural bias against actually doing anything meaningful about our health, and health care – in a culture built on fast-food and big-box store instant gratification, we're not the planet's most efficient planners of anything, with the possible exception of wars.

Add those two things together, and you have a medical establishment that can treat the hell out of your Stage IV cancer, extending your life for possibly years. Which sounds great until you see the impact that Stage II has on your life, and the costs associated with even early-stage treatment. I've seen what Stage IV treatment looks like. I've watched friends and acquaintances deal with that stage of various cancers – if I had Stage IV, I'd do whatever it takes, too, so don't misunderstand me here – and it's hell on wheels.

Draconian Stage IV treatments only give you around 10% survivability, in most cases, if you're diagnosed at Stage IV.

Cancer For Christmas

As I was writing this book, my copy of Wired magazine arrived, with a cover article by deputy editor Thomas Goetz titled, Cancer and the New Science of Early Detection. Stopped me in my tracks, and I've read the article front to back several times. A former executive at Cisco, Don Listwin, watched his mother die of ovarian cancer in 2001 after she had been misdiagnosed several times as having a bladder infection. Listwin left Cisco after his mother died, and in 2004 started the Canary Foundation, which is funding research into early detection.

There's a dearth of foundations funding research on early detection – most are focused on cures. A laudable goal, but what about the folks who wind up with the disease – cancer of any sort – before a cure is found? Without early detection, those getting Stage IV nasty-grams, the test results that basically tell you not to buy the family size tube of toothpaste because you likely won't live to squeeze it dry, will continue to increase.

One way to make an impact on organizations like the American Cancer Society and the National Cancer Institute, the leaders in cancer research, is to encourage them to shift their efforts to discovering better ways to detect cancer early. Cures will be great – in the meantime, early detection will save lives now.

That's the early detection lesson.

Doctors Aren't Gods – Not Even Close

Let's look at lesson #2, that the medical community needs to revamp its 'I'm Parnassus, you're just the patient' problem.

There's a reason it's called the practice of medicine – all doctors are still practicing. I don't mean for that to sound snarky...much. I think that over the centuries that medicine has been viewed as a 'calling', some doctors have misunderstood their place in the doctor/patient relationship. We're customers. We're not worshipers, nor are we lesser beings because we don't have MD behind our names. I suggest that each and every doctor on the planet invest in some Customer Relationship Management (CRM) training, for themselves and their staffs.

I've gotten great care from the doctors I worked with to defeat the Cancer Troll – even Dr. Drive-by and Dr. Surgeon Ego didn't actively try to kill me. Every single person's body is different, which makes it a challenge to diagnose anything beyond the common cold or a compound leg fracture.

In fact, what appears to be a cold can sometimes be the warning signs of lung cancer, and a leg fracture can be a symptom of metastasized bone cancer.

I'm not trying to be a fear-monger. My goal with this book is to encourage you to take care of your own journey through medical care. The doctors are doing the best they can, but if you don't ask questions, and don't answer theirs fully, you won't get the best, or in some cases even the right, care.

Remember, you're the customer

Doctors can often practice while looking behind them to see if the lawyers are coming. Combine doctors with lawyers. Stir in some patients who didn't get the results they wanted. Shake silly. Hey-presto, tort litigation!

I'm not saying that doctors are idiots – very, very few are. Tort lawyers may sometimes be over-enthusiastic about suing the pants off of everything in their path, but there are people who have suffered irreparable harm at the hands of doctors who either should have known better, or should not been licensed to practice medicine on anything, not even family pets.

The medical profession needs to follow the Hippocratic oath – first, do no harm - as an organization, and make sure it heals itself. Doctors who do a bad job don't do it in a vacuum – other doctors see the aftermath of their 'work'. Doctors who have no business touching patients, either because they're incompetent, or sadists, or both, should be run out of the profession on a rail. By other doctors, not by tort litigators representing damaged, or dead, patients.

Patients need to realize that doctors are not gods, in spite of the attitude that some doctors project (like Dr. Drive-by). Enter into your relationship with any doctor recognizing that you're at least 50% of the treatment plan – the customer, remember? - particularly if you're fighting a dangerous disease. Ask questions, and listen to the answers. If you don't like the answers, find a new doctor. Don't chew up the entire Yellow Pages in the process, but get a second opinion. Even a third, if necessary. Then pick a treatment plan, and get started.

And keep asking questions.

Another area that could us a lot of improvement is the technology of medical care. It flummoxes me that an industry that routinely uses cutting edge technology in care delivery – in imaging, in surgery, in medication, in monitoring – can't get their **** together on electronic medical records.

How crazy is it that every single doctor you visit requires you to fill out the same set of forms? Why can't we just have everything on a flash drive, present it at the desk when we check in, and then pick it up again on the way out? One of these days that will be a reality. I'm really looking forward to that day.

A true revolution would be for every single patient in the US to have his or her records online, with enough security to keep HIPAA happy. This is an idea that is completely achievable with current open-source software tools, that the army of brilliant geeks in the rapidly expanding open-source software development field could set up pretty efficiently.

Cancer For Christmas

A system like that would allow doctors to have a patient's records at their fingertips, and the ability to add new treatment reports and update patient statistics. Patients would be able to see their records, and track both progress and possible errors. Sounds like win-win to me, so how about we all work to make it happen?

Medical Insurance Is a Pyramid Scheme

OK, on to #3, My Opinion On Medical Insurance for $1000, Alex.

What I can do, for myself and for everyone else who needs medical care, particularly for any 'really big disease', is to add my voice to the discussion about how we manage healthcare here in the U.S.

Personally, I think it's crazy.

We have a culture that celebrates the hot new thing, whether it's an under-dressed flavor-of-the-month pop tart or a new drug with a great marketing campaign.

Can you say 'Viagra'? In fact, there was an under-dressed pop tart in an ad for Viagra a few years back. Britney Spears and Bob Dole in tied-in ads for Pepsi, alluding to Viagra, during the Oscars in 2001. Who could forget that high point in advertising?

This means that patients arrive in doctors' offices with those 'ask your doctor about...' brochures, which they've been encouraged to do by their televisions.

Developing a new drug takes many millions of dollars, and a wall-to-wall media campaign takes millions more. Getting a prescription for that drug means that somebody's gonna pay – if you've got prescription drug coverage, you don't directly, but your insurer does. Which means ultimately, you do pay. No coverage, and you find out quickly just how much name-brand drugs can add to your monthly budget. You wind up paying one way or the other.

New diagnostic tests and equipment come with equally high costs. If you stub your toe, do you really need an MRI? Yet I think there are times when that's exactly what happens, either because a patient demands it, or a doctor orders it because he's afraid he might get sued if he doesn't.

Drug companies send armies of sales reps out across the globe, into doctors' offices and medical centers, dropping off samples and singing the praises of their revolutionary new drug, what ever it is. Farmers don't do that, yet I think a lot of disease could be prevented, or managed, by eating better food. I recommend Michael Pollan's brilliant book, *The Omnivore's Dilemma*, if you'd like to know more about both where your food is coming from, and how to manage your food decisions with both your health and the health of your community in mind.

Cancer For Christmas

I think I really did find the man behind the curtain next to the Great & Powerful Oz known as the medical insurance industry. As I mentioned in my blog post dated Dec. 15, 2008, the medical insurance sector's gift to us all, 'managed care', has managed to insert a vast array of unseen people into the relationships between patients and doctors.

When managed care first hit the scene, I thought it sounded like a great idea. I learned very quickly that it was aimed at creating a relationship between patients' wallets and the insurer-backed HMOs, not between patients and doctors. I joined an HMO in 1980, and lasted for about 26 months. Once I found a doctor I liked – and I was only going for annual Pap smears and the occasional minor medical complaint at the time, since I was still in my 20s – I'd never see him or her again. When I called for my next appointment, the doctor would have left the HMO, and I'd have to start another search for a doctor that I felt comfortable with.

That was a warning sign that the process wasn't set up for doctors – if doctors don't stay in an HMO, that's got to mean something, right? It wasn't set up for patients, either – in addition to the doctor-doctor-who's-my-new-doctor game, it was also a Byzantine bureaucracy that made it difficult to get records, to find out lab results, or to even ask a question.

If the system isn't set up for doctors, and it isn't set up for patients, then who is it set up for? I'll give you three guesses. I bet you'll get it in one.

Think about every doctor's office you visit – think of how many administrative personnel they've got. At least 40% of the administrative cost of running a medical practice today is managing insurance claims. Every insurer has different forms, difference criteria for submission, and different payment systems. Some of them routinely deny every claim the first go-round, meaning that the entire claims process is extended by at least 100% in time and administrative cost.

Doctors may have made the big bucks back inna day, but those days are gone for most medical practitioners. The ones that still do make the big bucks are likely plastic surgeons with a largely discretionary, self-paid patient roster. In the cancer game – oncologists, surgeons, radiologists, pathologists – there is a large population of patients with Medicare, which has a very low payment schedule.

While the national dialogue over what's going to happen with medical care and health insurance in the U.S. continues over the next few years, as President Obama and his cabinet start to try to unravel the rat's nest that managed care has created, I've got some suggestions for how you can take ownership of your own health, if not your own health care.

Cancer For Christmas

Know what your family history is. Know what your risk factors are. Get screened for breast cancer and cervical cancer if you're female. Guys, get a regular PSA test after 50. All of us should get a colonoscopy at 50. I did, and I'm on the 10-year plan – with one dance with the Cancer Troll on my dance card, I'm going to be vigilant about regular screenings.

For which I will be paying out of my own pocket for the foreseeable future.

A dance with the Cancer Troll does a number on your insurance rates, which I'm sure doesn't surprise you. It didn't surprise me. What did surprise me:

Even without cancer, or any other red flags on your medical history, a woman will typically pay at least 20%, possibly as much as 35%, more in premiums than men for the same individual health insurance coverage. The reasoning, which I just love: women actually use the health care system. Men tend to use denial as their first line of defense against disease.

If you have cancer on your record within the last five years, and you can even get insurance, which is not guaranteed, it's likely to cost you over $1,000.00/per month and have a high deductible, possibly as high as $5,000.00. That's more than $17,000.00 down the well every year, with high co-pays if you've got 100% coverage, or low co-pays with what they call "80% co-insurance". Translated, that's your premiums, your deductible, your co-pays, and 20% of total cost of care. Ouch.

One option if you find yourself in this position is discount plans, offered at premiums ranging from $150 to $400 per month, that give you negotiated rates at doctors in their Preferred Provider Organization (PPO). They don't offer soup-to-healing-cancer-in-your-nuts coverage, particularly when it comes to hospitalization, but they do offer plans that let you see a doctor for around $30, get lab and imaging tests for around $150, and some hospitalization coverage, up to $60,000.00 in some cases.

I don't see medical discount plans as a global solution to handling medical care coverage. It leaves you exposed to high costs should the 'really big disease' – cancer, multiple sclerosis, ALS, Parkinson's, et al – become a part of your life. Discount plans can help you bridge the gap between no-coverage and real medical insurance, and you might find that they take care of your needs well. Just be aware that you're always one diagnosis away from financial disaster.

That's also true if you have medical insurance. Almost all medical insurance plans have a lifetime cap, usually around $1,000,000.00. That sounds like a lot until you come up against Stage III or Stage IV cancer, which can eat up $1M pretty quickly. What do you do then? Often, when you go over either an annual, or a lifetime, cap, you won't know it right away. You'll find out when the bills for a $2,000.00 PET scan or that last $20,000.00 hospital sojourn start to arrive.

Cancer For Christmas

Given that my insurer re-rated me in early December 2008 at around $1,200.00 per month with a $3,000.00 deductible, I'm looking into the discount plans I outlined before. What I'd most like is a consumer-driven plan – a high-deductible plan coupled with a Health Savings Account (HSA). Those are harder to find as an individual than as part of a group. As much as I like to fancy myself a rugged individualist, I'm hunting a group to join for just this reason.

A big expense I face monthly is the cost of my one-and-only regular prescription: Arimidex. This is one of the three AIs (the others are Femara and Aromisin) used to help post-menopausal women with hormone-positive breast cancer increase their 10-year survival odds. This tiny little pill is going to help me stay around for quite a bit longer, I hope. This tiny little pill also costs $500 per month. For 30 pills. Since AIs are relatively new drugs, there are no generics available in the US. Without insurance, that cost is almost as bad as the insurance premiums!

A medical discount plan can reduce that cost by 70% for a 90-day prescription, which would make it a much more affordable $150 per month. Or I could, if I chose to, switch to tamoxifen, the first breast-cancer prevention drug that hit the market in the 1980s. It's not as effective, but a generic is available. Time, and my wallet, will tell.

My central lesson-learned about medical insurance is that, by inserting themselves into every interaction a patient has with his or her doctor, and requiring that their labyrinthine administrative rules and regulations be followed to the letter for everything from dispensing an aspirin to signing off on a craniotomy, they do no good for doctors, and very little for patients.

Handing a third party the power to approve or deny medical care is, in my opinion, nuts. All it accomplishes is either delayed treatment, and sicker patients when treatment is finally delivered; or higher administrative costs across the board as actuaries, statisticians, and other non-medical personnel get their fingerprints on decisions that would be better made by the doctors and patients directly involved.

Of course, for this approach to be truly effective, the medical community has to police itself rigorously, as I suggested a few pages back. That has to happen before we can start extricating insurance companies from the doctor/patient relationship. I don't think it's an accident that the insurance industry is on both sides of this question: medical insurance, and medical malpractice insurance. If one side of that equation can be rendered moot by the medical community refusing to tolerate incompetence in its ranks, the other side, medical insurance, should reap some serious benefit. That may be naïveté on my part...but I don't think it is.

Your Health Is YOUR Responsibility

That's "What I Learned" #4.

The rising tide of medical costs, in the U.S. and other developed nations, can be laid at the door of our own individual unwillingness to take charge of our health by cutting back on drive-thru nutrition and doing what our TVs tell us to do: Eat this! Drink this! Who cares if it's loaded with sodium, saturated fat, and sugar! You deserve it!

We eat it, and drink it, usually while sitting in our cars or beached on our sofas in front of the TV. Which tells us about all the other stuff we're supposed to be eating, drinking, and buying.

It doesn't help that the television also tells you to 'ask your doctor about' everything from Cialis to drugs for schizophrenia. I think a schizophrenic has enough voices in his or her head that it's cruel and unusual that we'd add the television's, don't you?

I love a good meal. I enjoy a nice glass of wine. I really like all my electronic toys. The key is understanding why you want something – if you start with wanting to be healthy, that will inform your choices about what you'll let your TV tell you to do.

I made an illuminating discovery early in my journey, before I even had a firm diagnosis. As I was waiting for my magnification mammogram films to be processed back on Dec. 13, 2007, I read a chart on the wall in the exam room. It listed the risk factors for breast cancer, some of which were new to me:

Previous breast cancer (knew that)

Getting older (knew that, didn't know that 55 was a magic number - screw the golden years, right?)

Direct family history (I thought I'd caught a break here – I'm Patient Zero in my family)

BRCA1 and BRCA2 gene (knew that - still don't know if that's in play)

Not having kids (knew that)

Started menstruation before age 12 (did NOT know that, I got my period at 11)

Weight (knew that - menopause was not kind to me, nor was my surrender to my salt-and-grease addiction)

Alcohol (knew that, still enjoy my Vitamin W – wine – once or twice a week)

Hormone replacement therapy (knew that, won't be taking it)

Birth control pills might increase risk (was on them for a decade in my 20s – could have been a factor, or not)

When it's all added up, I hit the medium-to-high risk zone when I turned 55, thanks to the early periods, menopausal weight gain, and that 55th birthday. Sure enough, my next mammogram put me on the Cancer Troll's dance card. Be advised that a decade or more of clean mammograms does not mean you can slack off. I had fourteen of the suckers before I finally won the booby prize. Of all the risk factors, getting older and family history are the two you can do the least about.

Cancer For Christmas

What risk factors do you have for cancer, heart disease, and other life-threatening diseases? As you get older, those risk factors gather more steam, just as my turning-55 booby prize proved. Smoking, bad nutrition, a lack of exercise can all add to your ticket in the genetic lottery and wind up giving you some sort of unwanted prize. Knowledge is power, baby – denial just makes knowing more painful, because then the knowledge can come too late.

I'm actively working on ditching at least a majority of the weight I gained as a side-benefit of menopause. Down around fifty pounds so far, with another forty to go. I also, after decades of smoking, managed to quit for good and all a few years ago. I know I'm still at risk for lung cancer, but I'll keep my fingers crossed and pay attention to my lungs by using them often and well at the gym and on my bike.

There's not a lot I can do about getting older – particularly since I love life enough that I'm in no hurry to leave. There's not much I can do about random chance, which I think plays as much a part in finding oneself winding up with a cancer diagnosis as family history does.

What we all can do, as a nation, and as members of the human race, is to start demanding more from medicine. Medical vendors - big pharma and medical equipment manufacturers - and the medical insurance industry have been driving the bus for a while now, and it looks like the wheels are coming off.

Doctors and hospitals are pursued relentlessly by drug companies and medical equipment manufacturers, with samples and blandishments of all kinds, all aimed at driving up the number of prescriptions for whatever this week's wonder drug might be, or diagnostic procedures of questionable value but high billable cost.

The medical insurers are the brain-trust that gave us managed care, where unseen hands have the power to grant, or deny, medical treatment. All of those unseen hands are attached to humans who draw salaries, which I firmly believe add to the overall cost of both medical insurance premiums and medical care.

Access to medical care is a basic human right. However, medical care is not, nor can it be, free. Somebody pays, whether you pay 100% of your medical costs out of your own pocket, have great insurance, or are relying on Medicare or Medicaid. The challenge we face, as a nation and as a global community, is to figure out how to meet those costs.

Medicare is often used as an example of how a national single-payer plan would work.

I'm sorry, but that sounds like a nightmare worse than the nightmare we're already having. I don't see how turning over the health care of an entire nation to an almost-bankrupt bureaucracy that's nearly Soviet in its size and un-workability is any kind of solution.

Cancer For Christmas

In an article on Slate.com in April 2008, Mark Gimein pointed the finger directly at the American health care consumer for the high cost of health care. I have to say that I think he's at least 75% right. Doctors, hospitals, and medical insurers all have a part to play in the tragi-comic opera that healthcare has become. The U.S. spends 16% of its national income on health care, yet still has a lower life expectancy than most developed countries.

How about we try this: as consumers, how about we start taking some steps on our own behalf?

Each of us needs to take some kind of meaningful action to ensure our own health: better nutrition, and at least some exercise. Just because you can heat it up in the microwave in under 5 minutes doesn't mean you should eat it every day. Start reading labels, and if you can't say it, don't eat it. Stop smoking, start walking. Stop listening to your television when it tells you to buy stuff. Who's in control of your life: you, or Sara Lee?

As far as ensuring, and insuring, our health goes, there's a new President being sworn in on Jan. 20, 2008. One of the central planks in his platform was tackling the mess that is the medical care and insurance system in the U.S.

Let's all weigh in on that work, and help get all of us moving toward better health, better medical care, and better ways to manage the costs of both.

That's my story, and I'm stickin' to it.

The Gift

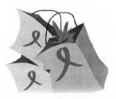

*The opportunity to share all this with you –
I treasure your attention, and am eternally
grateful for it!*

Cancer For Christmas

If you're diagnosed with breast cancer, the first book you should get your hands on is Dr. Susan Love's Breast Book, by Susan M. Love, M.D., with Karen Lindsey. It's got so much information in it that it verges on too much information. However, when it comes to your health, is there any such thing as too much information?

BreastCancer.org has a wealth of information about breast cancer diagnosis and treatment, as well as a wide variety of expert Q&A and community forums. (www.breastcancer.org)

Breast cancer advocacy organizations that I recommend are the grandmother of them all, the Susan G. Komen Foundation, www.komen.org, and my personal favorite breast cancer advocacy group, Save the Tatas – great name and great t-shirts. www.savethetatas.org.

Great information on cancer of any type can be found at the web home of the American Cancer Society: www.cancer.org.

Information on clinical trials for cancers of all types is available from the National Cancer Institute: www.cancer.gov.

Every kind of cancer, as well as every type of life-threatening and/or chronic disease, has its own advocacy group, with its own website. Consult Dr.

Google, he knows and reveals all. Be careful, though, to make sure the information is coming from a reliable medical source, not "Fred's Miracle Woo-Woo Cancer Cure Page".

There's a lot of really bad information – woo-woo – out there on the Wild Wild Web. Make sure you're getting information from a knowledgeable source, which means don't get medical advice from someone who's not a medical professional.

Caveat emptor, baby.

Speaking of the Doctor, here are some nuggets of wisdom that Dr. Google led me to:

Neutropenia:

Chemotherapy-induced neutropenia: risks, consequences, and new directions for its management.

Crawford J, Dale DC, Lyman GH., Divisions of Oncology and Hematology, Duke University Medical Center

Cytotoxic chemotherapy suppresses the hematopoietic system, impairing host protective mechanisms and limiting the doses of chemotherapy that can be tolerated.
Neutropenia, the most serious hematologic toxicity, is associated with the risk of life-threatening infections as well as chemotherapy dose reductions and delays that

may compromise treatment outcomes. The authors reviewed the recent literature to provide an update on research in chemotherapy-induced neutropenia and its complications and impact, and they discuss the implications of this work for improving the management of patients with cancer who are treated with myelosuppressive chemotherapy.

Despite its importance as the primary dose-limiting toxicity of chemotherapy, much concerning neutropenia and its consequences and impact remains unknown. Recent surveys indicate that neutropenia remains a prevalent problem associated with substantial morbidity, mortality, and costs. Much research has sought to identify risk factors that may predispose patients to neutropenic complications, including febrile neutropenia, in an effort to predict better which patients are at risk and to use preventive strategies, such as prophylactic colony-stimulating factors, more cost-effectively.

Neutropenic complications associated with myelosuppressive chemotherapy are a significant cause of morbidity and mortality, possibly compromised treatment outcomes, and excess healthcare costs. Research in quantifying the risk of neutropenic complications may make it possible in the near future to target patients at greater risk with appropriate preventive strategies, thereby maximizing the benefits and minimizing the costs. Copyright 2003 American Cancer Society.

[Source: http://www.ncbi.nlm.nih.gov/
pubmed/14716755,]

Chemotherapy-induced neutropenia is a condition characterized by abnormally low blood levels of infection-fighting neutrophils, a specific kind of white blood cell. The most common reason that cancer patients experience neutropenia is as a side effect of chemotherapy. Chemotherapy involves the use of drugs to destroy cancer cells. Chemotherapy works by destroying cells that grow rapidly, a characteristic of cancer cells. Unfortunately, chemotherapy also affects normal cells that grow rapidly, such as blood cells in the bone marrow, cells in the hair follicles, or cells in the mouth and intestines. Chemotherapy-induced neutropenia typically occurs 3–7 days following administration of chemotherapy and continues for several days before neutrophil levels return to normal. The type and dose of chemotherapy affects how low the neutrophil count drops and how long it will take to recover.

Chemotherapy-induced neutropenia is important because it may: Increase a patient's risk of life-threatening infection and/ or disrupt delivery of cancer treatment, resulting in a change to the planned dose and time. The fewer the neutrophils in the blood and the longer patients remain without enough neutrophils, the more susceptible patients are to developing a bacterial or fungal infection. Neutrophils are a major component of antibacterial defense mechanisms. As the neutrophil count falls below 1.0, 0.5, and 0.1 x 109/L, the frequency of life-threatening infection rises steeply from 10% to 19% and 28%, respectively. If patients develop a fever during neutropenia they may require treatment with intravenous antibiotics and admission to the hospital until the number of neutrophils in the blood returns to sufficient levels to fight the infection.

Another reason neutropenia is important is that, in some cases, it can be severe enough that it can cause the chemotherapy treatment to be delayed or dose reduced, which reduces some patients' chance for cure. When patients are treated with chemotherapy, it is for the purpose of destroying cancer cells in order to reduce symptoms from your cancer, prolong your survival or increase your chance of cure. The dose and time schedule of chemotherapy drugs administered have been scientifically determined to produce the best chance of survival or cure. If patients develop neutropenia, doctors may have to delay your treatment or reduce the doses of chemotherapy until the neutrophil counts have recovered. Clinical studies have shown that, for certain cancers, reducing the dose of chemotherapy or lengthening the time between treatments lowers cure rates compared to full-dose, on-time treatment. There are however strategies for the prevention of chemotherapy-induced neutropenia that have been proven to reduce the incidence of fever, infection, admission to the hospital and allow patients to receive treatment on schedule.

Risk factors

Who is at a higher risk for chemotherapy-induced neutropenia? Patients receiving chemotherapy that decreases the number of white blood cells.

Patients who already have a low white blood cell count, or who have previously received chemotherapy or radiation treatment.
Patients age 70 and older who may be at risk of more severe infection and longer hospitalizations

Patients with other conditions affecting their immune system.

Prevention
Chemotherapy-induced neutropenia can be prevented in most patients with the use of white blood cell growth factors. Blood cell growth factors are naturally occurring substances called cytokines that regulate certain critical functions in the body. They are responsible for stimulating cells in the bone marrow to produce more blood cells. The white blood cell growth factors approved by the U.S. Food and Drug Administration for the prevention of chemotherapy-induced neutropenia are Neupogen (filgrastim) and Neulasta (pegfilgrastim).
[Source: http://en.wikipedia.org/wiki/Chemotherapy-induced_neutropenia,]

Casey here again - If what you've read above scares the **** out of you, good. Start eating plenty of red, orange, and dark green vegetables and fruits, even if you're not undergoing chemotherapy. Here's why I made that decision:

Cancer For Christmas

Immune-Boosting Foods
If you were to look at a sample of your blood under a microscope, you would see an enormous number of red blood cells whose job is to carry oxygen to your body tissues. Here and there among them are white blood cells of various kinds, and they are the key soldiers that make up your immune system. When abnormal cells arise in the body, it is white blood cells' job to recognize and eliminate them.

Some white blood cells are able to engulf and destroy abnormal cells—including cancer cells—as well as viruses, bacteria, and other invaders. Other white blood cells facilitate this process in various ways, for example, by producing antibodies, protein molecules that attach to foreign or abnormal cells and flag them for destruction.

The immune system is critically important in fighting cancer. Individual cancer cells can arise in all of us from time to time. Cancer cells can also break free from an existing tumor and spread to other parts of the body. If your immune system is vigilant, it recognizes and destroys cancer cells before they can take hold. So strengthening the immune system is a key strategy in cancer prevention and survival.

Foods That Boost Immunity
Like soldiers anywhere, your immune cells fight more effectively when they are well nourished. Certain nutrients have been shown to be immune boosters.

Beta-carotene.
Beta-carotene is an important antioxidant. It also boosts immune function.

The best sources are orange and yellow vegetables and fruits, such as carrots, yams, and cantaloupes, as well as green, leafy vegetables. Research has shown that beta-carotene supplements are not necessarily as safe or effective as food-derived beta-carotene.

The U.S. Government does not have a specific recommended intake for beta-carotene, except to say that 11 milligrams per day for men and 9 milligrams per day for women will give you your daily dose of vitamin A (beta-carotene is converted to vitamin A in the body). Research studies generally use somewhat higher intakes and have shown that the amount of beta-carotene in two large carrots (about 30 milligrams) consumed daily has a measurable immune boosting effect.

Vitamin C.
Nobel Laureate Linus Pauling was a strong advocate for vitamin C, and research suggests that, indeed, vitamin C boosts immunity, in addition to its antioxidant abilities. Once again, vegetables and fruits are the preferred sources. The recommended daily intake is only 90 milligrams per day for men and 75 milligrams per day for women. However, some researchers have recommended higher amounts, typically in the form of supplements and usually in the

neighborhood of 500 to 2,000 milligrams. There appear to be no adverse effects from these higher doses of vitamin C.

Vitamin E.
When it comes to vitamin E, a little is good, but a lot is not necessarily better. Researchers have found that individuals eating vitamin E-rich foods such as barley, pumpkin, and sunflower seeds tend to have improved immunity. But increasing vitamin E intake to high levels through supplements can impair immune function.
The best advice appears to be to stick with food sources and avoid vitamin E supplements.

Zinc.
The mineral zinc has been promoted for its cold-fighting abilities, and, indeed, it works. However, when it comes to zinc or any other mineral, you want neither too little nor too much, just as with vitamin E.

Researchers in New Jersey discovered this fact accidentally. They tested zinc's effects in a group of older men and women. Some were given zinc tablets, while others got placebo tablets that looked and tasted just like zinc. And to make sure that everyone was generally well-nourished, the researchers also asked everyone to take a daily multiple vitamin. When the researchers later checked their immune function, they found, to their surprise, that everyone had an immune boost. You can guess why. The multiple vitamin apparently counteracted a variety of mild nutritional deficiencies, and that improved their immunity.

However, the researchers had a second, and more surprising finding: The volunteers taking as little as 15 milligrams of zinc actually had worse immune function than those who got placebos.

In other words, zinc is an essential nutrient and a helpful immune booster when ingested in minute quantities. But it is easy to go overboard, and excess zinc interferes with immune function. The recommended amount of zinc in the daily diet is 8 milligrams for adult women and 11 milligrams for adult men.

[CASEY NOTE: Good sources of zinc are beef, lamb, turkey, and salmon.]

[Source: http://www.cancerproject.org/resources/ handbook/section7.pdf]

Lentanin

This extract from the Shiitake mushroom has been in use for almost thirty years. It has been successfully employed against a variety of tumors in laboratory animals. Lentanin has been used, like so many immune modulators, to protect against the side effects of chemotherapeutic agents. The combination has been found effective in stomach, colorectal, and breast cancers (K. Okuyama, et al, Cancer, 1985 and T. Taguchi, 1983)

[Source: http://www.scribd.com/doc/11645812/The-Cancer-Solution-by-Dr-ROBERT-E-WILLNER-MD-PhD }

The April 2008 Slate.com article by Mark Gimein – his opinion about what's really driving up health care costs:
http://www.slate.com/id/2190273/pagenum/all/#p2

And the January '09 cover story in Wired, by Thomas Goetz, Why Early Detection Is the Best Way to Beat Cancer:
http://www.wired.com/medtech/health/magazine/17-01/ff_cancer

Whatever you find yourself dealing with medically, be indefatigable about asking questions, getting the best information, and evaluating your choices.

Your life is in your hands.